STRUCTURED EXERCISES in STRESS MANAGEMENT

A WHOLE PERSON™ HANDBOOK
FOR TRAINERS, EDUCATORS AND GROUP LEADERS

VOLUME I

edited by
Nancy Loving Tubesing, EdD
and
Donald A Tubesing, MDiv, PhD

Whole Person Press

Library of Congress Catalog Card Number: 83–61073
ISBN: 0–938586–01–7

REPRODUCTION POLICY

Unless otherwise noted, materials that appear in this book may be freely reproduced for small-scale (fewer than 100 copies per year) education/training activities. For such uses no special permission is required. However, the following statement must appear on all reproductions:

Reproduced from **Structured Exercises In Stress Management, Volume 1,** Nancy Loving Tubesing and Donald A Tubesing, Editors. © 1983 Whole Person Press, PO Box 3151, Duluth MN 55803.

Large-scale (more that 100 copies per year) reproduction, or inclusion of any material from this book in other publications for sale or widespread distribution, is prohibited without prior written permission from Whole Person Press.

For further information please write for our Permissions Guidelines and Standard Permissions Form. Permission requests must be submitted at least 30 days in advance of your scheduled printing or reproduction.

Printed in the United States of America by Port Cities Printing, Superior WI

10 9 8

Published by: **WHOLE PERSON PRESS**
1702 E Jefferson St
PO Box 3151
Duluth MN 55803
218/728-6807

PREFACE

With the publication of this volume and its companion, **Structured Exercises in Wellness Promotion, Volume 1,** *we proudly inaugurate our new line of topical Whole Person HANDBOOKS.*

The Whole Person HANDBOOKS are specially designed for trainers, consultants, counselors, teachers, adult education specialists, nurses, psychologists, clergy, managers, group workers, health educators — for anyone using the experiential approach to learning. Each HANDBOOK contains a compilation of the best structured exercises for teaching wellness promotion or stress management, with complete instructions for your use. We've personally tested all of these processes in a variety of settings and believe that nowhere will you find a collection of more effective structured experiences for actively involving the participant — as a whole person — in the learning process.

As you will soon discover, many of these exercises we've designed ourselves and refined them in the more than 1,000 workshops we've conducted during the past 10 years. Some are new combinations of time-tested group process activities. Others were submitted by people like you who continually strive to add the creative touch in their teaching. Whenever we've been aware of the source of an idea, we've noted it.

Please note our policy for reproduction of HANDBOOK contents. Our purpose in publishing these volumes is to foster inter-professional networking and to provide a framework through which we can all share our most effective ideas with each other. The layout is designed for easy photocopying of worksheets and training notes.

☞ *Feel free to adapt and duplicate any sections of the Handbook for your use in training or educational events—* **as long as you use the proper citation as indicated on the facing page.**

☞ *However, all materials are still covered by copyright. Prior written permission from Whole Person Press is required if you plan large scale reproduction or distribution of any portion of the HANDBOOK. If you wish to include any material in another publication for sale, please send us your request and proposal.*

We are grateful to the many creative trainers who have so generously shared their "best" with you in these HANDBOOKS. Why not return the favor? We encourage you to submit your favorite structured exercises for inclusion in future Volumes. Do let us know what works well for you so that we can carry on the tradition of providing a forum for the exchange of innovative teaching designs.

Duluth MN　　　　　　　　　　　　　　　*Nancy Loving Tubesing*
April 1983　　　　　　　　　　　　　　　　*Donald A Tubesing*

WHOLE PERSON ASSOCIATES INC
consultants and publishers

**specialists in stress and wellness
programs with a whole person focus**

PUBLISHING

• stress and wellness handbook series •
for trainers, educators and group leaders
• innovative training materials, tape and workbook packages •
• unique "workshop-in-a-book" self-help guides •
• practical "workshop-in-a-box" audio and video tape programs •
• unusual relaxation tapes •
• health-related educational games •

CONTINUING EDUCATION

• workshops, inservice training, keynote speeches, conferences •
stress management, burnout, communication
wellness/high vitality, self-care
• professional organizations, community-based helping agencies •
hospitals, business, government, education, civic groups

PRODUCT DEVELOPMENT

• research and development •
wellness-oriented products for health-conscious organizations
• design of creative stress management premiums/promotions •
for employees, clients, customers

CONSULTATION

• development and implementation •
stress management and wellness programs
for clients around the world
• curriculum design •
• creative problem solving •
• interdisciplinary think tank •

TABLE OF CONTENTS

ACTION PLANNING

GROUP ENERGIZERS

INTRODUCTION

Stress is a fact of life — and from the board room to the emergency room to the living room people are searching for ways to manage stress more positively.

Structured Exercises in Stress Management, Volume 1 offers you 36 designs you can use for helping people move beyond information to implementation. Each exercise is structured to creatively involve people in the learning process, whatever the setting and time constraints, whatever the sophistication of the audience. To aid you in the selection of appropriate exercises, they are grouped into six broad categories:

Icebreakers: These short (10–20 minutes) and lively exercises are designed to introduce people to each other and to the subject of stress management. Try combining an icebreaker with an exercise from the assessment or management section for an instant evening program.

Stress Assessments: These exercises explore the symptoms, sources and dynamics of stress. All five processes help people examine the impact of stress in their lives. You'll find a mixture of shorter assessments (30–60 minutes) and major theme developers (60–90 minutes). Any exercise can easily be contracted or expanded to fit your purpose.

Management Strategies: Each of these five processes explores the issue of overall strategies for dealing with the stress of life. Participants evaluate their strengths and weaknesses and identify skills for future development.

Skill Developers: Each volume in this handbook series will focus on a few coping skills in more depth. The four exercises in this section highlight relaxation, surrender, laughter and interpersonal contact skills.

Action Planning/Closure: These four exercises help participants draw together their insights and determine the actions they wish to take on their own behalf. Some also suggest rituals that bring closure to the group process.

Energizers: The twelve energizers are designed to perk up the group whenever fatigue sets in. Sprinkle them throughout your program to illustrate skills or concepts. Try one for a change of pace — everyone's juices (including yours!) will be flowing again in 5–10 minutes.

The HANDBOOK format is designed for easy use. You'll find that each exercise is described completely, including: *goals, group size, time frame, materials needed, step-by-step process instructions, and variations.*

🖙 *Special instructions for the trainer and scripts to be read to the group are typed in italics.*

✔ Questions to ask the group are preceded by a check.

➤ Directions for group activities are indicated by an arrow.

● Mini-lecture notes are preceded by a bullet.

Although the processes are primarily described for large group (25 to 100 people) workshop settings, most of the exercises work just as well with small groups, and many are appropriate for individual therapy or personal reflection.

If you are teaching in the workshop or large group setting, we believe that the use of small discussion groups is the most potent learning structure available to you. We've found that groups of four persons each provide ample "air time" and a good variety of interaction. If possible, let groups meet together two or three different times during the learning experience before forming new groups.

These personal "sharing groups" allow people to make positive contact with each other and encourage them to personalize their experience in depth. On evaluations, some people will say "Drop this," others will say, "Give us more small group time," but most will report that the time you give them to share with each other becomes the heart of the workshop.

If you are working with an intact group of 12 people or less, you may want to keep the whole group together for process and discussion time rather than divide into the suggested four or six person groups.

Each trainer has personal strengths, biases, pet concepts and processes. We expect and encourage you to expand and modify what you find here to accommodate your style. Adjust the exercises as you see fit. Bring these designs to life for your participants by inserting your own content and examples into your teaching. Experiment!

And when you come up with something new, let us know . . .

ICEBREAKERS

1 INTRODUCTIONS 2 (p 1)
These three creative icebreakers quickly involve participants in exploring stress through personal history, current journalism, and object identification. (10-30 minutes)

2 RELAXATION BINGO (p 5)
This mixer helps participants get acquainted by finding others who regularly practice specific relaxation techniques. (10-20 minutes)

3 CLEAR THE DECK! (p 7)
In this guided group fantasy participants mentally identify worries/concerns that are occupying their minds and set them aside so they can be fully present. (10-15 minutes)

4 TWO MINUTE DRILL (p 10)
Participants pair up and answer a series of four questions about stress as many times as possible in two minutes. This quick theme expander gets everyone involved and helps people focus on the topic. (10-15 minutes)

5 STRESS BREAKS (p 13)
Participants brainstorm favorite "quickie stress reducers" and select the best for random use as stress breaks during the remainder of the learning experience. (15 minutes)

6 PERSONAL STRESSORS AND COPERS (p 15)
Participants identify current life stress and discover a wealth of coping strategies used by their neighbors. This brief warm-up exercise can easily be expanded into a major theme presentation. (20-30 minutes)

1 INTRODUCTIONS 2

These three creative icebreakers quickly involve participants in exploring stress through personal history (**Life Windows**), current journalism (**Stress Collage**), and object identification (**Rummage Sale**).

GOALS
To get acquainted.

To discover personal themes of stress and coping.

To promote non-linear exploration of stress-related issues.

GROUP SIZE
Unlimited

TIME FRAME
10–30 minutes

MATERIALS NEEDED
Life Windows: a blank sheet of paper for each participant.

Stress Collage: a sheet of newsprint for each participant; old newsprint and magazines; tape or glue; magic markers scattered throughout the group.

Rummage Sale: an assortment of objects.

PROCESS

LIFE WINDOWS

☞ *With more than 20 participants, the trainer will need to form smaller groups (3–12 people) for introductions. The larger the groups, the more time will be needed.*

1) The trainer distributes blank paper to all and demonstrates as she asks participants to fold the paper in half lengthwise and then in half again crosswise. When people open the paper flat again, there should be creases in the form of a cross dividing

the page into four sections. The trainer instructs participants to label the boxes *childhood* (top left box), *teens* (top right box), *adult* (bottom left), and *future* (bottom right).

2) Participants are instructed to think back into their childhood and identify one or two particularly stressful events that occurred for them during that period. The trainer directs participants to use the *childhood* box to write down a brief description of the stressful event or events they have recalled.

3) After everyone has identified a stressful childhood experience, the trainer asks people to focus on the coping strategies they used during that time period and make a note of two or three favorite childhood copers (e.g. pouting, temper tantrums, acting "cute," imaginary playmates, etc).

4) The trainer next asks participants to focus on their teen-age years, noting briefly in the *teens* box a stressful experience or two and a few adolescent era coping techniques (e.g. listen to stereo, hot-rodding, drinking, etc).

5) Next participants reflect on the stresses and strains of their adult life, noting one or two particular events in the bottom left-hand box. The trainer asks them to think about their coping patterns as adults and identify two or three techniques that they frequently use.

6) The last box is for the future. The trainer asks people to imagine ahead to a life experience they anticipate will be stressful. After writing that event in the *future* box, participants identify two or three coping techniques they would like to develop more fully before that event occurs.

7) Participants pair up and describe the stress/coping patterns of their life window to their partners.

STRESS COLLAGE

☞ *This exercise works best when participants have plenty of space to spread out. Tables are nice, but the floor will do if people are dressed informally.*

1) The trainer gives each participant a sheet of blank newsprint and places stacks of newspapers and magazines, glue, tape, and magic markers at strategic locations around the room.

2) Participants are instructed to make a stress collage using photos, advertisements, news stories, headlines, cartoons, handwritten comments, etc (10 minutes).

3) The finished collages are posted around the room and participants take a few minutes to tour the "gallery" before returning to their seats.

4) The trainer chooses one collage and says to the group, "I'd like to know this person better." The designer of the collage stands, introduces himself and explains one significant item from the collage. This person then chooses another collage and asks for an introduction.

5) This procedure continues until all participants have introduced themselves.

VARIATIONS

■ If the group is large, the trainer can divide participants into smaller groups (4–12) for the collage descriptions and introductions.

■ If the group is small, everyone could gather around the chosen collage while its designer introduces herself. The whole group would then move to the next collage until all are introduced.

RUMMAGE SALE

☞ *This exercise works best with less than 20 participants. The trainer will need to assemble a diverse collection of objects in advance (at least twice as many items as participants). Include the commonplace (dishrag, wrench, envelope, key ring, toilet paper, rag doll, rock, paperclip, apple, cough drop, etc). Place the items on a table and cover them with a sheet until the exercise has been explained.*

1) The trainer briefly describes the exercise to participants, indicating this will be an opportunity to discover something about themselves and to get acquainted with others in the group.

2) The trainer uncovers the table full of objects and invites participants to wander around the table studying the objects and noting which ones appeal to them. After checking them out

at leisure, participants are to choose one object that symbolizes or reminds them of one or more of their current stressors.

3) As soon as participants find their "stress object" they remove it from the table and take it back to their seat with them.

4) When everyone is settled, the trainer invites people to introduce themselves to the whole group by showing their chosen object, describing why they made the choice and telling how the object symbolizes their stress.

VARIATIONS

■ For a larger group, limit the objects to 30. People choose one item but don't take it. Instead they write down their choice along with the reasons for their selection. Participants introduce themselves by describing the object fully to the group and disclosing what it represents to them.

■ Instead of identifying objects with current stressors, participants could instead choose an item that represents their coping style. This variation could be used as a closure/planning exercise with participants picking an object that reminds them of a resolution they want to implement or a stress management strategy they want to develop more fully.

TRAINER'S NOTES

2 RELAXATION BINGO

This mixer helps participants get acquainted by finding others who regularly practice specific relaxation techniques.

GOALS
To give an overview of suggestions for tension reduction.

To facilitate discussion of relaxation activities.

GROUP SIZE
Best with groups of 15–50 persons

TIME FRAME
10–20 minutes

MATERIALS NEEDED
Relaxation Bingo worksheets for all participants.

PROCESS
1) The trainer distributes the Bingo sheets and instructs participants to circulate leisurely in the group, asking each other about the tension-relieving activities they enjoy. Emphasis should be on making contact and sharing information rather than completing all items on the sheet (10–15 minutes).

2) The trainer may want to reconvene the group as a whole and ask participants to discuss what they learned about each other and new ideas for relaxation.

TRAINER'S NOTES
Submitted by Martha Belknap

RELAXATION BINGO

Find someone here who participates in these activities regularly as a means of relaxation. Ask them to sign their names in the appropriate boxes. Try to find a different person for each activity. Fill in the center square with *your* favorite relaxation activity.

plays a musical instrument or sings	spends time in the woods, mountains, desert or beach	uses a hot tub, hot springs, steam-room, or sauna	rides a bike or motorcycle for pleasure	keeps a journal, diary, or dream notebook
practices a martial art	takes naps or sunbaths	works in the yard or garden	runs, jogs, or takes long walks	plays with young children or animals
does deep breathing exercises	meditates regularly	your favorite	eats only natural, healthy food	spends leisure time in the park
enjoys a snow or water sport	goes hiking or camping	enjoys a craft or manual hobby	enjoys an aerobic sport	listens to quiet music
practices dancing or gymnastics	attends theatre, concerts, shows	reads a lot for pleasure	gets and/or gives massages	practices yoga

3 CLEAR THE DECK!

In this guided group fantasy participants mentally identify worries/concerns that are occupying their minds and set them aside so they can be fully present.

GOALS

To prepare participants for the learning session.

To teach a tension-reducing technique that can be used in anxiety provoking situations.

To expose participants to the potency of fantasy and visualization.

GROUP SIZE

Unlimited; works well with individuals, too.

TIME FRAME

10–15 minutes

PROCESS

1) The trainer makes a few comments about our incredibly active minds and the difficulty most people have shifting gears. We hold on to the concerns, worries and feelings of one situation even while we're already launched into the next. He explains that his brief fantasy exercise should help participants let go of some of their mental preoccupations so that they can be fully present in the learning situation.

2) Participants are instructed to find a comfortable position with feet on the floor and eyes closed. The trainer asks people to relax, take a deep breath and turn their attention inward.

3) After a few collective deep breaths, the trainer slowly reads the **Clear the Deck Guided Fantasy** script.

   ☞ *The trainer will need to personalize the script, inserting his own examples and the parameters of the specific learning situation. Slow yourself down, too! Read slowly and pause at the ellipses (. . .) to allow participants to experience their images.*

©1983 Whole Person Press PO Box 3151 Duluth MN 55812   (218) 728-6807

4) As participants return their attention to the room, the trainer can ask for comments, observations, insights. Most people are surprised that they have the power to *decide* not to worry for a time. The trainer may want to raise questions like, "What was your box like? What did you put in it? When would this technique be especially helpful to you?"

VARIATIONS

■ After the fantasy experience participants could divide into small groups to process the fantasy. Add 10–15 minutes to the time frame.

TRAINER'S NOTES

Submitted by Gloria Singer

©1983 Whole Person Press PO Box 3151 Duluth MN 55812   (218) 728-6807

CLEAR THE DECK GUIDED FANTASY SCRIPT

I'd like you to take a few minutes to focus on the various concerns, preoccupations, worries that you have brought with you today (to this class, workshop, etc) . . . There may be any number of things that are on your mind — whether you remembered to unplug the coffee pot before you left the house this morning, the unfinished conversation that you had with someone . . . the errands that you need to run when you leave here . . . the project at (work/school) that's due tomorrow . . . plans you're making for the weekend . . .

So take a moment to really focus on what these concerns are for you — develop a mental list . . .

To the extent that these concerns are occupying your thoughts — making claims on your energy — you are not able to be Fully Present, here and now for this experience . . .

Probably, there is nothing that you can do during the next (____ minutes/hours) about these concerns, except to worry . . . and that will distract you from all you can be learning here . . . So let's put those worries away for a while . . .

I'd like you to create in your mind a box . . . with a lid on it . . . and a lock and a key . . . The box can be any size and shape . . . but it needs to be large enough and strong enough to hold all the concerns you've identified . . . So take a moment to visualize this box as clearly as you can . . . The box is before you now, with the lid open . . .

Now I'd like you to put each of your concerns in the box, one-by-one . . . don't forget any now . . . and as you are doing this, tell yourself, "There is nothing I can do about this for now . . . and so I'm going to put this concern away in a safe and secure box — for now — while I'm here, and I know I can come back later, and reclaim all of my concerns. . . "

Now when you've put all your preoccupations and concerns in the box, I'd like you to close the lid and lock it with your key . . . Now I'd like you to put your key in your pocket or someplace else for safekeeping . . . and I'd like to remind you that at the end of this experience, you can unlock your box and pick up whre you left off . . .

And when you're ready, I'd like you to slowly open your eyes and come back here . . .

4 TWO MINUTE DRILL

Participants pair up and answer a series of four questions about stress as many times as possible in two minutes. This quick theme expander gets everyone involved and helps people focus on the topic.

GOALS

To generate personal sharing about stress patterns.

To discover subconscious attitudes, goals, and motivators.

GROUP SIZE

Unlimited; easily adapted for work with individuals.

TIME FRAME

10–15 minutes

MATERIALS NEEDED

Newsprint posters with two minute drill questions.

PROCESS

1) The trainer asks participants to find a partner who was born in a different month from them.

2) Once everyone is paired up, the trainer instructs them to designate one partner as *Cadillac* and the other as *Volkswagon* (or any other descriptive pairing — apples and oranges, nights and days, ins and outs, ups and comings, cats and dogs, etc — whatever might be fun for the group).

3) The trainer explains the next step to the group as follows:

> ➤ In just a minute I'm going to have you turn and face each other and the *Cadillacs* are going to ask a series of questions which the *Volkswagons* will answer. The *Cadillacs* will begin by asking these four questions one at a time:
> > 1) How do you keep yourself stressed?
> > 2) What do you get from it — positively and negatively?
> > 3) What do you really want?
> > 4) How could you create that?

➤ After two minutes you'll switch roles. I call this a two minute drill and it will give you an opportunity to get to know one another.

4) The trainer posts the four questions at several spots around the room so that all participants can easily refer to them, and then continues with the instructions:

➤ *Cadillacs*, listen carefully to the responses and when your *Volkswagon* partner has answered all four questions, go back and ask the same four questions over again — and again — as many times as possible in two minutes. I'll keep time.

➤ *Volkswagons*, don't think too long about your answers — your immediate reactions will probably be valid and revealing. Try to restate the question as part of your answer — "I keep myself stressed by . . . ," etc. You'll probably want to answer the first question differently each time — which will also change your other answers. The idea is to come up with as much information as possible in two minutes. Take some risks. Let yourself go with the flow.

➤ *Cadillacs* — I'd really like you to encourage your partners by listening intently, making eye contact, nodding, and keeping them on track.

5) The trainer demonstrates the technique, asking a nearby *Cadillac* to pose the questions and then answering them honestly and openly herself, repeating the question as part of the answer (eg, "I keep myself stressed by . . . ," I really want . . . ," etc). Once the trainer has modeled, she instructs participants to turn and face their partners, get as close together as is comfortable, look into each others' eyes, and begin with the *Cadillacs* asking question 1.

☞ *For maximum effectiveness, participants should be seated knee to knee for this exercise, with feet flat on the floor, hands comfortably in the lap. If space or furniture does not permit this posture, the exercise may be done standing.*

The trainer may add a little zip to the process by blowing a whistle to begin the drill and again at the two minute marks. This works especially well with very large groups.

6) After two minutes the trainer gives a signal and asks participants to switch roles. This time the *Volkswagon* ask the four questions and the *Cadillacs* answer.

©1983 Whole Person Press PO Box 3151 Duluth MN 55812   (218) 728-6807

7) After two minutes the trainer stops the group and asks partners to talk with each other about what they learned or what the experience was like for them.

8) The trainer may gather the entire group and ask for insights and observations.

VARIATIONS

■ This exercise can be infinitely varied by changing the questions according to the specific topic under discussion, the needs of the group, and the trainer's inclinations. One of these sequences could be substituted —

✔ What do you appreciate about yourself?

✔ In what ways would you like others to appreciate you?

✔ How do you sabotage that?

✔ How could you get appreciation?

✔ What games do you play?

✔ What do you get from it?

✔ How do you hide in your role?

✔ What do you hide?

✔ What do you get from that?

✔ What would be different if you didn't hide?

■ Or the trainer may suggest a single question to be answered over and over for two minutes:

✔ I feel loved when ...

✔ I cope by ...

■ Instead of asking one partner to pose the questions for the other to answer, the trainer could direct participants to respond to the questions without prompting. The questions could be translated into unfinished sentences and posted around the room or handed out as a worksheet.

Submitted by J J Cochran who adapted it from an exercise she learned from the Insight Training Program, Los Angeles, CA.

©1983 Whole Person Press PO Box 3151 Duluth MN 55812   (218) 728-6807

5 STRESS BREAKS

Participants brainstorm favorite "quickie stress reducers" and select the best for random use as stress breaks during the remainder of the learning experience.

GOALS

To affirm personal coping strategies.

To generate a list of diverse ideas for reducing stress and relieving tension.

To get acquainted.

GROUP SIZE

Unlimited

TIME FRAME

15 minutes brainstorming; 2–5 minutes for each break.

MATERIALS NEEDED

3x5 note cards (4 for each participant)

PROCESS

1) The trainer distributes four note cards to each participant and asks them to think about the various ways they use to relieve tension or short-circuit the stress response. What quick tricks do they use to unwind or unstress themselves? Participants should focus on all the little stress breaks (5 minutes or less) they may take during the day and jot down 5 or 10 or 20 on one of the note cards.

   ☞ *The trainer will want to give several examples of typical stress breaks such as a cup of coffee, a deep breath, a quick smoke, putting your feet up, taking a walk, etc, as well as some lively, creative options such as screaming in an empty elevator, a vigorous tooth brushing, yoga, whistling, counting paperclips, an erotic daydream, needlepoint.*

---

2) Participants pair up with a neighbor and discuss their personal self-care strategies for stressful times or situations. (3–5 minutes)

3) The trainer asks participants to think about their partner's stress break suggestions and choose the three most intriguing, creative, fun ideas. After identifying their favorite three, they should write them down — one on each of the remaining 3x5 cards. If the stress break is not self-explanatory, participants should write brief instructions for how to do it.

> ☞ *The trainer can give examples again with brief instructions (eg, polite yawn — yawn keeping lips close, etc). He may need to repeat the instruction that participants are to write down stress breaks described by their partners.*

4) The trainer collects all the 3x5 cards and places them in a container at the front of the room. He then asks someone to draw one card out of the reservoir and leads the group in doing the stress break written on the card.

> ☞ *Even if the chosen idea seems absurd or impossible in the classroom setting, do it anyway. Be creative! Pantomime the activity. Modify it. Do it in miniature. Have fun!*

5) At appropriate times during the remainder of the learning experience (at least once an hour) the trainer stops for a stress break, repeating *Step 4.*

> ☞ *If the exercises are brief, the trainer may want to try two or more at each break time.*

6) The trainer (or someone from the group) may want to make a compilation of all the suggestions from the cards, duplicate it, and distribute the complete list to all participants.

VARIATION

■ In *Step 2* participants could divide into groups of 3, 4, 5 or 6 people to discuss their stress break ideas. Each group lists the ideas on newsprint and then brainstorms together on other ways to unstress yourself. These lists are posted around the room and consulted at "stress break times" when each group in turn picks a technique and leads the whole group in the chosen process. Add 5–10 minutes.

Thanks to Linda Nowobielski who was the catalyst for this exercise.

©1983 Whole Person Press PO Box 3151 Duluth MN 55812   (218) 728-6807

6 STRESSORS AND COPERS

Participants identify current life stress and discover a wealth of coping strategies used by their neighbors. This brief warm-up exercise can easily be expanded into a major theme presentation.

GOALS

To generate a personal and group list of stressors.

To identify typical coping strategies and generate a list of potential skills for dealing with stress.

GROUP SIZE

Unlimited

TIME FRAME

20–30 minutes

MATERIALS NEEDED

Blackboard or newsprint easel with markers.

PROCESS

1) The trainer asks participants to make a list of their current stress — all the big and little things that nag, worry, upset or drain them in their life right now — all the situations on and off the job that are currently stressful. (2–3 minutes)

   ☞ *The trainer should give a variety of examples such as a sick child, conflict with a co-worker, financial worries, a hangover, uncomfortable chairs, pending divorce, etc.*

2) Participants pair up with a neighbor and share their lists. After two minutes, the trainer asks each pair to choose one stressor they have in common and one that is unique to each partner.

3) The trainer suggests that participants might want to get a sense of what stresses others bring with them to the group. The trainer invites each pair to share their chosen common and unique stressors with the group at large. The trainer writes down all of the stressors on the blackboard or newsprint.

   ☞ *The trainer may want to stop here and spend some time teaching about stress and stressors. Or she may group the stressors as she writes them on the board for use in a later discussion.*

4) The trainer asks participants to change their focus of attention from the problem to the solution. She asks people to make a second list — this time writing down their favorite coping techniques. Participants are to note the typical ways they deal with this or other stress in their lives. (2–3 minutes)

☞ *The trainer will need to give several examples of coping techniques (eg, smoking, talking to a friend, a hot bath, problem-solving, exercise, drinking, getting organized) and encourage people to list several that they use frequently.*

5) Participants pair up with a different neighbor and compare notes on coping. After two minutes the trainer asks them to choose one skill they have in common and one coping strategy unique to each partner.

6) The trainer reconvenes the group and comments on the wealth of coping resources represented by all the individuals in the room. She asks for volunteers to share the skills they had in common with their partners and writes them down on the blackboard.

7) After several examples have been given, the trainer asks all participants to share in turn one of their unique coping skills. The only trick is that each person must name a skill that has not been previously mentioned. As the coping strategies are identified, the trainer writes them on the board and comments on the richness and diversity of skills suggested by the "coping experts" in the room.

☞ *The trainer may want to group the skills according to some overall strategies or stop and elaborate on some. Inevitably some people will mention "negative" copers. This is a perfect opportunity to talk about the costs and benefits of different coping strategies. This exercise provides an excellent prelude to an in-depth discussion of coping strategies.*

VARIATION

■ To focus on stress in the workplace the trainer can ask participants to list only work-related stress and on-the-job coping techniques. All other instructions remain the same.

STRESS ASSESSMENTS

7 STRESS SYMPTOM INVENTORY (p 17)

In this whole person assessment of stress exhaustion symptoms participants look at their distress patterns and identify issues they want to work on during the course. (30-40 minutes)

8 THE JUGGLING ACT (p 21)

In this novel stress assessment participants inventory their stressors and recall the impact of stress on their internal and external environments. (40-60 minutes)

9 STRESSFUL OCCUPATIONS CONTEST (p 28)

Participants divide into occupational groups, brainstorm on- the-job stressors and campaign to have theirs declared the "most stressful occupation." This lively exercise is particularly effective for mixed professional groups or in a setting that includes personnel from various job status levels. (35-45 minutes)

10 STRESS RISK FACTORS (p 32)

In this assessment/chalktalk exercise participants reflect on their personal stress "at-risk-level" by examining their overall lifestyle patterns. (10-20 minutes)

11 LIFETRAP 1: WORKAHOLISM (p 37)

This extended, multi-process exercise allows participants to explore the meaning of work in their life. Participants check themselves against the symptoms of the "Hurry Sickness" that signals the onset of workaholism. They examine the results of this stress-laden lifestyle as well as the belief system that undergirds it. (60-90 minutes)

7 STRESS SYMPTOM INVENTORY

In this whole person assessment of stress exhaustion symptoms participants look at their distress patterns and identify issues they want to work on during the course.

GOALS

To identify symptoms of stress exhaustion in all areas of life.

To target specific symptoms for change.

To articulate personal goals for the learning experience.

GROUP SIZE

Unlimited; also effective for work with individuals.

TIME FRAME

30–40 minutes

MATERIALS NEEDED

Stress Exhaustion Symptoms worksheet for each participant.

PROCESS

1) The trainer briefly introduces the exercise, pointing out that stress affects us as whole people, so we're likely to experience symptoms of stress exhaustion not only in our bodies — but also in our emotional reactions, our mental state, our relationships with others and our spiritual life.

2) The trainer distributes the **Stress Exhaustion Symptoms** worksheet and asks participants to check any symptoms they've noticed lately, and to add any of their symptoms that aren't on the list.

   ☞ *The trainer may want to elaborate further on the symptom list. Alert participants that there may be other underlying causes of any of these symptoms that should be checked out, but underscore that this list represents common stress-related complaints.*

3) Once everyone has completed the checklist, the trainer directs participants to look over their identified symptoms and circle

those that cause them most concern. Which ones are they worried about right now?

4) Next the trainer asks participants to review the entire list of symptoms again and put a star by any symptom that would be a real signal of distress to them.

> ☞ *The issue here is individual meaning systems and motivation. The trainer may want to ask the questions more directly: "Which of these symptoms, if it occurred in your life, would you certainly pay attention to and be motivated to change the stressful pattern that caused it?"*

5) The trainer asks participants to reflect for a moment on the patterns they see in their stress symptoms. Are most of their symptoms in one area? Are they more concerned about physical symptoms than spiritual ones? Are any areas symptom-free? Participants jot down notes an any insights/observations.

6) The trainer invites participants to explore their symptoms further by drawing a picture of their symptom collection on the back of the worksheet. No one has to be a Picasso — people can have fun using words, symbols, stick figures, diagrams or whatever to convey an overall perspective of their stress exhaustion symptoms. (5 minutes)

> ☞ *Allow plenty of time here for people to get their creative juices flowing. Some groups will need lots of permission and encouragement to play around with their drawing.*

The trainer asks people to fill in the blanks and write these sentences somewhere on their worksheet:

➤ Right now I'm concerned about, _____, _____, _____.

➤ During this course I'd like to work on _____, _____, _____.

7) Participants divide into groups of four or rejoin their small sharing groups. Each person takes a few minutes to describe his picture to the group and share the symptoms that cause him most concern and the issues he wants to work on. (15–20 minutes)

8) The trainer reconvenes the group and asks for observations/ insights/comments.

☞ *This exercise should be followed with a skill assessment development process that participants can apply to the symptoms they have targeted as troublesome.*

VARIATIONS

- Rather than draw a picture in *Step 6* the trainer could ask people to write a dialogue with one or more of the symptoms they identified as being of particular concern. Participants will probably need some guidance at first (eg, "Write it like a play," "Start with the symptom talking to you and then answer back.")

- For a brief (10–15 min) assessment to precede an in-depth exploration of sources of stress, drop *Steps 6 and 7.*

TRAINER'S NOTES

STRESS EXHAUSTION SYMPTOMS

Check the symptoms of stress exhaustion you've noticed lately in yourself.

PHYSICAL
__ appetite change
__ headaches
__ tension
__ fatigue
__ insomnia
__ weight change
__ colds
__ muscle aches
__ digestive upsets
__ pounding heart
__ accident prone
__ teeth grinding
__ rash
__ restlessness
__ foot-tapping
__ finger-drumming
__ increased drug,
alcohol, tobacco use

EMOTIONAL
__ anxiety
__ frustration
__ the "blues"
__ mood swings
__ bad temper
__ nightmares
__ crying spells
__ irritability
__ "no one cares"
__ depression
__ nervous laughter
__ worrying
__ easily discouraged
__ little joy

SPIRITUAL
__ emptiness
__ loss of meaning
__ doubt
__ unforgiving
__ martyrdom
__ looking for magic
__ loss of direction
__ cynicism
__ apathy
__ needing to
"prove" self

MENTAL
__ forgetfulness
__ dull senses
__ low productivity
__ negative attitude
__ confusion
__ lethargy
__ whirling mind
__ no new ideas
__ boredom
__ spacing out
__ negative self-talk
__ poor
concentration

RELATIONAL
__ isolation
__ intolerance
__ resentment
__ loneliness
__ lashing out
__ hiding
__ clamming up
__ lowered sex drive
__ nagging
__ distrust
__ lack of intimacy
__ using people
__ fewer contacts with
friends

©1983 Whole Person Press PO Box 3151 Duluth MN 55812   (218) 728-6807

8 THE JUGGLING ACT

In this novel stress assessment participants inventory their stressors and recall the impact of stress on their internal and external environments.

GOALS

To identify stressors and assess personal stress level.

To explore the impact of stress on the body.

To determine the effects of stress.

GROUP SIZE

Unlimited

TIME FRAME

40–60 minutes

MATERIALS NEEDED

Blackboard or newsprint easel; a copy of the **Juggling Act Inventory** for each participant.

PROCESS

1) The trainer briefly introduces the exercise and then distributes the **Juggling Act Inventory**.

2) The trainer asks participants to pretend that the juggler on the worksheet represents them and the balls symbolize all the stressors and strains that they're juggling in their lives right now.

   The trainer instructs participants to label each ball — in the air and on the ground — with one of their stressors.

   ☞ *The trainer will need to allow ample time for participants to get focused. If people seem to be having difficulty identifying stressors, prompt the group by giving some examples or asking, "What people, feelings, situations, problems, changes, pressures, etc are causing stress in your life right now? How about at work? Or at home?"*

The trainer may encourage people to add balls if there aren't enough to depict their current stress level.

3) Once everyone has filled in their balls, the trainer asks them to reflect on their drawing and jot some notes in response to these questions:

✔ How do you feel about the number of balls you're juggling in your life? Too many? Too much stress? Not enough? Just right?

✔ What about the balls on the ground? Did you choose to let them fall or did they drop by default?

✔ Look at each ball separately. How do you feel about it? Is it something you want to continue juggling? Is it something you can control or modify? What goodies do you get from keeping this one in the air? What distress does it cause you?

☞ *The trainer will need to adjust the pacing of questions to the group. Allow plenty of time for people to reflect and write, but don't drag this part out waiting for the last person to finish.*

4) Next the trainer invites participants to consider the physical dimension of their stress and to indicate inside the juggler's figure what are their personal body signals and symptoms of stress.

☞ *The trainer may want to give several examples such as the racing pulse, tense muscles and rapid breathing of the immediate stress response as well as the headache, hypertension or colitis that indicate long range stress effects.*

Participants are encouraged to use words, symbols, shadings, pictures to embellish their figure in response to these questions:

✔ How does your body feel when you're under stress?

✔ What parts of your body signal stress and tension in you?

5) After everyone has had a chance to identify the internal consequences of their stress, the trainer asks them to shift their focus to the external consequences. Participants use the empty spaces on their worksheets to record the non-physical effects of their stress on them as whole persons. The trainer asks:

✔ How else are you affected by stress? What other results do you see in your attitudes? Your feelings? Your relationships with family? Your interactions at work? Your creativity or productivity? How does your stress level impact you and the people and situations around you?

☞ *The trainer may want to give examples such as "always fighting with my husband," "lose my temper easily," "can't make contact with friends," "no time for the kids," etc.*

6) The trainer builds a group composite stress picture in three columns on the board. First she solicits examples of stress situations that guarantee a stress reaction for participants. Then she asks for typical body signals and symptoms of stress. Finally she invites illustrations of the non-physical results of stress in people's lives.

☞ *During this step, the trainer needs to keep the tempo moving quickly, stopping occasionally to make a point about stress and encouraging interaction among participants.*

7) The trainer elaborates on the data generated by the group in a chalk talk covering basic stress concepts. The trainer will probably want to include some or all of the following issues:

- **Stress is universal**. Everyone experiences it every day. You're all exposed to environmental stress such as crowding or ragweed pollen or extreme temperatures or noise pollution. Any change that forces you to adapt is bound to produce stress. So will physical exertion or danger.

- **Perception is a common source of stress**. You encounter a situation that *appears* threatening, so you activate the stress response just as if the danger were physical and life-threatening rather than just embarrassing or emotionally painful. You hear a siren and see a flashing red light — panic time! A friend or relative disapproves of your behavior — stress attack! You have to telephone a customer and apologize for a delay or mistake — adrenalin overload!

- Stress may also come from your own negative **feelings or bad habits**.

- **Stress is not all bad**. Everyone needs it! The stress response protects us and mobilizes us in time of real physical danger. Stress also adds flavor and zest to life. It motivates us to try new things, to accomplish our life tasks, to reach our goals.

- **Too much stress can be distressing** — and eventually disastrous. It may have a detrimental effect on your physical health, your emotional stability, your relationships with people, your sense of purpose in life.

● The line between the **eustress** that turns you on and the **distress** that wears you out is often difficult to distinguish. The point is not to eliminate stress, but to find the level that's right for you.

● **Healthful stress levels vary greatly** from individual to individual. Your optimal level will be different from that of your friends and family. A guitar has six strings, each of a different size and under a different amount of tension. An E string plays best at a certain tension level. The A string requires a different level. Tighten either one too much and it snaps. Loosen it too far and you can't make music. You need to find the amount of tension that helps you play your own beautiful music.

● How will you distinguish eustress from distress in your own life? Learn to know your signals of stress overload (or underload). And when you notice one — take action!

Listen to your body! It will let you know when you've had "enough" — listen to that queasy stomach or stiff neck or bout of insomnia.

Listen to your feelings, too. When moments of enjoyment and peace are rare and your moods are as unpredictable as the weather, you may have reached your stress quotient.

Listen to your spirit — apathy, cynicism and loss of meaning are often symptoms of stress overload.

Listen to your relationships. When your irritability index goes up, it's probably time to turn the stress level down.

8) Participants divide into groups of four and describe their inventory pictures to one another, focusing particularly on any new insights they discovered. (15 minutes)

9) The trainer reconvenes the group and asks for comments/observations/insights before leading participants in a stretching or relaxation routine to close the exercise.

VARIATIONS

■ To make a comprehensive 90-minute stress management presentation, the trainer could precede this exercise with an icebreaker, insert a group energizer or two and follow-up with a skills assessment and brief planning process.

TRAINER'S NOTES

Submitted by Sally Strosahl

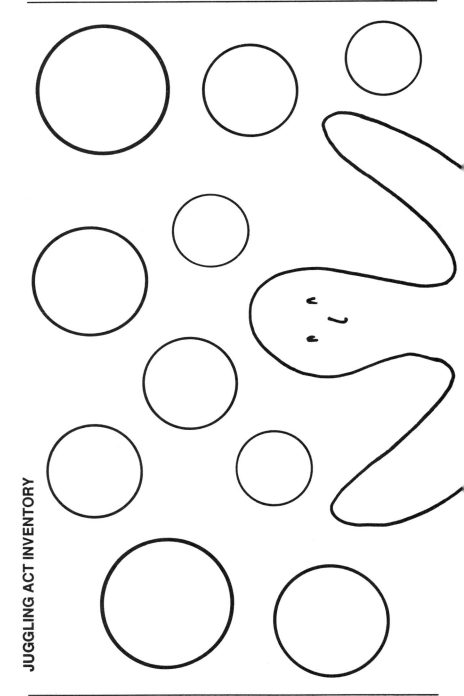

JUGGLING ACT INVENTORY

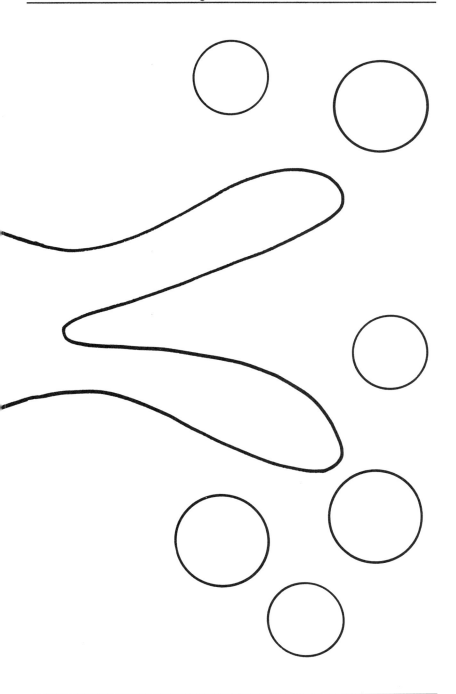

9 STRESSFUL OCCUPATIONS

Participants divide into occupational groups, brainstorm on-the-job stressors and campaign to have theirs declared the "most stressful occupation." This lively exercise is particularly effective for mixed professional groups or in a setting that includes personnel from various job status levels.

GOALS

To heighten awareness of job related stressors.

To explore the typical stresses of a variety of occupations.

To encourage creativity and humor.

GROUP SIZE

Unlimited; works best with 20 or more people.

TIME FRAME

35–45 minutes

MATERIALS NEEDED

Blackboard or newsprint easel; blank paper for each participant; simple prizes.

PROCESS

☞ *Process instructions assume the group includes participants from several different professions. See the variations for suggestions on adapting the design for other group compositions.*

1) The trainer polls the group to discover the variety of occupations represented by participants. He writes the occupational groups on the board.

2) The trainer asks participants to list two or three stressors they feel are particularly related to their job or occupation. He then asks for examples of stressors for each of the occupations and writes them on the board.

🖙 *This is just a brief overview. Three or four stressors for each job is plenty. Keep the pace moving rapidly.*

3) The trainer briefly introduces the issue of job-related stress; including the following points in his presentation.

- Every occupation has its stress. From the tedium of the assembly line to the tension of the operating room to the pressure of professional athletics. Whatever your job — some stress is bound to come with the territory.

  Many occupations claim to be the ***most stressful*** — including secretaries, air traffic controllers and presidents!

  🖙 *The trainer may want to include here the 1978 ranking of most stressful occupations by the National Institute for Occupational Safety and Health: 1) laborer; 2) secretary; 3) inspector; 4) lab technician; 5) office manager; 6) foreman; 7) manager/administrator; 8) waiter/waitress; 9) machine operator; 10) farmer.*

- In this exercise we're going to take a closer look at the typical stresses of your occupation, and how stressful that job is in comparison to others represented here.

4) The trainer designates areas in the room for each occupation and directs participants to move to the place that corresponds most closely to their own job description.

   🖙 *The trainer may need to combine some similar occupations or divide a large job grouping in order to achieve groups of optimal size (3–6 persons).*

5) Once everyone has relocated and settled down, the trainer outlines the group task.

   ➤ Each group is to spend the next 15 minutes brainstorming a list of the stresses inherent in their occupation and formulate a strategy for convincing other participants that theirs is the most stressful occupation.

   ➤ After 15 minutes, the whole group will be reconvened and each group will be allowed 2 minutes to make their presentation. The presentation can take the form of a skit, a dialogue, a speech, a debate — whatever the group can devise.

   ➤ On the basis of these presentations, participants will decide the winners of the **Most Stressful Occupation Contest**.

6) The trainer directs the groups to get started and encourages them to use their creativity and to include all members in the

planning and presentation. The trainer announces the time at 5 minute intervals to help the groups pace themselves.

7) After 15 minutes, the trainer reconvenes the group and explains the voting process. After each presentation participants are to rate the stress of the occupation on a scale from 1 (little stress) to 10 (very high stress).

8) The trainer asks for volunteers or randomly orders the groups for making presentations. After each presentation, the trainer reminds participants (including the presentors) to rate the stress level of that occupation.

9) When all groups have had their turn on the soap box, the trainer asks participants to look over their ratings and mark their 1st and 2nd choices for most stressful occupations. He then collects the ballots and tallies them on the board.

10) The trainer makes a humorous speech summarizing the contest results and awards appropriate prizes (eg, stresstabs, applause, group backrub, etc) to the three highest stress groups.

VARIATIONS

■ The trainer may choose several occupations/categories from the current ranking by the National Institute of Occupational Safety and Health as the focus for this exercise (eg, minister, retail sales clerk, professor, construction worker, telephone operator, plumber, bus driver, parent, etc).

Participants could be randomly assigned to occupational groups or allowed to choose their own as long as groups do not exceed six persons. Group rankings of the most stressful occupations could then be compared to the Institute's ranking.

■ If the trainer knows the group composition in advance, he can decide on occupational groupings based on the professions/positions represented.

■ When all participants come from the same organization, the list of stressful occupations could include all status and skill levels (eg, maintenance, security, clerical, supervisors, line staff, administrators, business managers, etc). In *Step 4* participants could be asked to join the group representing their own job specialty or to temporarily explore the occupational stress of a different role in the organization.

TRAINER'S NOTES

10 STRESS RISK FACTORS

In this assessment/chalktalk exercise participants reflect on their personal stress "at-risk level" by examining their overall lifestyle patterns.

GOALS

To help participants understand the long-term results of an over-stressed, high-risk lifestyle.

To demonstrate that isolated, traumatic, short-term stressors seldom cause major damage unless accompanied by a cluster of additional negative lifestyle elements.

To help participants distinguish between those stressors they can control and those they cannot.

GROUP SIZE

Unlimited; also effective in work with individuals.

TIME FRAME

10–20 minutes

MATERIALS NEEDED

Blackboard/newsprint easel, **Risk Factors in Stress Exhaustion** worksheets for all participants.

PROCESS

1) The trainer introduces the exercise by outlining the following concepts:

- Although most people tend to focus on the pain of their most immediate daily stressors, seldom are these the ones that wear us out and defeat us — we can tolerate trauma if it's temporary.

- **We human beings are resilient.** We can handle a lot without falling apart. In fact, that's the positive function of our stress reaction. It helps us rise to the occasion and get ourselves safely through even the roughest of times — at least temporarily.

- Stress exhaustion and the debilitating effects of stress are usually the result of a high-risk lifestyle, lived month after month, year after year. **It's the long-term drain that wears us out,** not the one "bad" month or even one "bad" year. No one stressor defeats us. We all handle a lot in our lifetime — all of us being scarred and wounded veterans of one thing or another. We don't necessarily fall apart in a crises.

- **No one lives a risk-free life.** Living a "high-risk" lifestyle does not guarantee that we will fall apart! — just as living a "low-risk" lifestyle does not guarantee that we will never fall apart. However, the odds for us or against us do, indeed, change according to the lifestyle we choose.

2) The trainer distributes the **Risk Factors in Stress Exhaustion** worksheet and asks participants to make note of those risk factors that are present in their currtent lifestyle choices.

   The trainer outlines the 10 stress risk factors on the board and expands each concept using the suggestions below. On the left column of the worksheet participants record whether or not each factor is contributing to their current *at risk status*.

   ☞ *For participants who balk at either/or choices, suggest some system for ranking the relative intensity of risk factors (eg, * to ***).*

   The trainer begins by asking *"How high a risk are you?"* and then goes on to describe the ten factors that increase your chance of stress exhaustion.

   - **Negative perception habits** — always looking at the gloomy side, "getting up on the wrong side of the bed" day after day.

   - **Family pressures** — they come in many forms and shapes. None of us in families escape their pressures, although sometimes they are more extreme than at other times.

   - **Environmental demands** — stressors beyond our control such as poor economy, bad weather, taxes, inflation.

   - **Work problems** — boring job, conflict with co-workers, too much pressure, worry, angry boss, etc.

   - **"Helper" mentality** — trying to respond to everyone else's needs all of the time. As admirable as this may be, it's also draining.

   - **Responsibility without authority or resources or gratitude** — a job to do, without permission to do it your way or a job to

©1983 Whole Person Press PO Box 3151 Duluth MN 55812   (218) 728-6807

do, without the wherewithal to get it done or a job to do, without any appreciation or thanks.

- **Negative coping patterns** — faulty stress safety valves (eg, alcohol consumption, overeating, pouting, temper tantrums, overwork). Relying on behaviors that work in the short run but are dead-end streets. Ultimately, they cause more problems than they solve.

- **Undeveloped stress management skills** — relying on the same style of coping for every problem (no flexibility). Relying on skills you were "born with", rather than exploring and learning more functional patterns (no growth).

- **Broken compass** — an internal guidance system gone haywire (no purpose, few goals, conflicting values, confused beliefs — out of touch with who you are and what's important to you).

- **Personal tragedy** — trauma and major life changes. We all face these, and alone they do not defeat us unless we already live under such risk that we have no resiliency left.

3) After having completed the list, the trainer reminds participants that no one factor breaks people, but the accumulated drain of carrying many risk factors over time wears down even the strongest person. Participants are asked to reflect on the level of risk they carry, based on the number of risk factors that are currently active in their lives.

4) The trainer points out that some risk factors are beyond individual control, while others are due directly to personal choices and can be removed from one's lifestyle if desired. Using the right hand margin of the worksheet, participants note which risk factors they could choose to avoid and which they simply must learn to live with.

5) Participants reflect in writing on (a) their current level of risk, (b) ways in which they could reduce their risk, and (c) any additional observations/insights/personal resolutions that occur to them.

6) The trainer asks participants to share comments and observations with the entire group.

©1983 Whole Person Press PO Box 3151 Duluth MN 55812   (218) 728-6807

VARIATIONS

- Enough data and insights are generated by this exercise that the trainer, if time permits, may divide the participants into smaller groups of 4–6 persons for sharing of observations and personal reactions. Small groups will add 15–20 minutes to the time requirements.

- This assessment/chalktalk may be combined with exercises that help participants analyze their current individual stressors (eg, *Personal Stressors and Copers,* p 15, and *The Juggling Act,* p 21). This combination should help participants not, able to comfortably handle

RISK FACTORS IN STRESS EXHAUSTION

Active in my life?

Can I do some- thing about it?

Yes	No		I can change	Have no control
		1) Negative perception habits.		
		2) Family pressures.		
		3) Environmental demands.		
		4) Work problems.		
		5) "Helper" mentality.		
		6) Responsibility without — authority, resources, or gratitude.		
		7) Negative coping patterns.		
		8) Undeveloped stress management skills.		
		9) Broken compass.		
		10) Personal tragedy.		
		TOTALS		

General observations/insights regarding my current risk level for stress exhaustion:

How could I reduce my risk level?

Resolutions?

11 LIFETRAP 1: WORKAHOLISM

This extended, multi-process exercise allows participants to explore the meaning of work in their life. Participants check themselves against the symptoms of the "Hurry Sickness" that signals the onset of workaholism. They examine the results of this stress-laden lifestyle as well as the belief system that undergirds it.

GOALS

To help participants explore the meaning and place of work in their lives.

To assist participants in identifying the life-eroding stress bred by a lifestyle of addiction to work.

To offer participants options for controlling and relieving the addiction to work.

GROUP SIZE

Unlimited

TIME FRAME

60–90 minutes

> ☞ *This is a complex subject and an extended exercise. It cannot be meaningfully completed in less than one hour.*

MATERIALS NEEDED

The Hurry Sickness Test and **Workaholic Belief Systems** worksheets for each participant.

PROCESS

A. WORKAHOLISM: STRESS-PRODUCING LIFETRAP (5–10 min)

1) The trainer introduces the issue of workaholism as a seductive lifetrap that's bound to produce stress. In this chalktalk section of the exercise, the trainer may want to cover most of the following concepts.

● **Work is important.** Accomplishments and success breed confidence and allow us to contribute in a positive manner to our world. Those who work hard and take their responsibilities seriously usually are rewarded for their efforts with both praise and promotions. Our culture admires people who produce — and for good reason!

● However, **hard work and success can become addictive.** For the work addict, personal worth becomes dependent upon how much one gets done and how successful one becomes. Fearing failure, addicts are *driven* to succeed. They feel compelled to move from one success to the next, faster and faster.

● **People who adopt this harried lifestyle create for themselves a life full of distress.** They accelerate their tempo — trying to do more and more in less and less time. They push themselves to accumulate possessions and status; they continually compete with others and with themselves. These are all symptoms of the workaholic disease "The Hurry-up Sickness."

● Doctors Rosenman and Friedman, California heart specialists, contend that people who "catch" the hurry-up sickness, which they nicknamed *Type A Behavior*, are 7 to 10 times more likely to develop heart disease than are their more relaxed counterparts.

● **They define Type A behavior as:** *a particular complex of personality traits including excessive competitive drive, aggressiveness, impatience, and a harrying sense of time urgency. Individuals displaying this pattern seem to be engaged in a chronic, ceaseless, and often fruitless struggle — with themselves, with others, with circumstances, with time, sometimes with life itself.*

● The results? Energetic, strong-willed persons, independent and capable, caught in a self-made "trap" of attempting to hold everything together, trying to achieve greater success, hoping to complete all dreams, going faster and faster, neglecting the poetic and personal side of life, are one day confronted with the question *"Has it been worth the price?"*

They awaken to well-earned heart disease or ulcers, to extra-marital affairs, to children gone delinquent, to cold-hearted dismissal from the company to which they "sold" their lives. They are victims of their own enlarged sense of duty gone haywire.

- Addicted "performers" usually **treat themselves like machines** and tend to drive themselves until they break down in one way or another.

B. EXPLORING THE WORK ADDICTION TRAP (15–25 min)

2) The trainer invites participants to explore how closely they fit into the workaholic pattern. He distributes a copy of **The Hurry Sickness Test** worksheet to each person and guides the group through a self-reflection process.

➤ First, assess yourself using the checklist of 14 behavior patterns typical of the workaholic, Type A personality.

➤ Next, take a look at the list of qualities describing one who is not addicted to work (labeled Type B) and consider how well they apply to you.

➤ Now it's time to take a stand. Based on these descriptions of Type A and Type B, judge your own level of addiction to work and place an "X" on the continuum at that spot.

➤ Take a minute now to list some of the behaviors and images that influenced your ranking of yourself as workaholic (Type A) and those specific behaviors and images that influenced you to think of yourself as non-addicted (Type B).

3) The trainer announces that the meeting room will be turned into a live human continuum. He designates a point on one wall to represent 100% Type A and a spot on the opposite wall to represent 100% Type B.

➤ Imagine a line drawn on the floor connecting these two points. This line is the Type A — Type B work addiction continuum. The middle of this line represents 50% Type A and 50% Type B, other percentages fit between the extremes and the middle.

➤ Now I'd like everyone get up and move to the spot on the continuum in the room that corresponds with the location of your "X" on the worksheet continuum.

☞ *Don't neglect the humor in this situation. Point out these "typical" patterns, and any others, that emerge in the process.*

+ *The "A's" hurried to their spots and are now drumming their fingers waiting for you "B's" to line up!*

+ *Often with spouses and friends in the room we hear a few remarks like, "You get over there where you belong."*

+ *The "A's" were placed away from the coffee lest they all charge to the front. This way the "B's" can get their coffee at leisure for once.*

+ *Looking at the "A's" the trainer may say, "Well, a prime characteristic of "A's" is that they see the addiction in themselves, but they each believe that they are the one in a hundred who can get away with it. I'm here to tell you that in this room, I'm the one!"*

C. SMALL GROUP SHARING AND DISCUSSION (20–30 min)

4) The trainer instructs the group to divide into small sharing groups of 4 persons each. Participants may be directed to consciously choose whether they want to be with people near them on the continuum or get together with others from the far ends of the continuum.

☞ *Again the trainer may joke about group consistency. Four Type A's will hold an energetic, task-oriented discussion, and it will be hard to get a word in edgewise. Type B groups may not ever get to the agenda but will probably pick a comfortable spot to meet, relax, get to know each other, and find some common ground.*

5) The trainer instructs group members one-by-one to take five minutes each for sharing whatever they wish about their work-related patterns and addictions and the stress that results. When all have had a turn groups may discuss similarities and differences, overall themes that emerged, etc.

6) The trainer reconvenes the entire group and asks for observations and insights from the small group discussions.

☞ *Sometimes an individual will argue that "this work addiction idea is all bunk." If she is too persistent, simply tell her you'd rather not compete right now, so she wins! Then move right along with the process.*

D. EXPLORATION OF THE ISSUES (20–25 minutes)

7) The trainer outlines from the whole person perspective the potential distress that may result from workaholism and the negative effects of this pattern.

- **Physical**: heart problems, hypertension, muscular tension, fatigue.

- **Intellectual**: diminished creativity, madly repeating the same pattern over and over with little time to explore new ideas.

- **Emotional**: emotions hurried, comfortable only with "tough" emotions, little tenderness; the child-like poet inside has no voice.

- **Social**: few close attachments, lack of intimacy; using people for what they can do, not who they are; loneliness.

- **Spiritual**: playing God — no acknowledgment of power beyond sold, no need for God, "I'll do it myself"; "things" are meaningful, money and success are worshipped; emptiness, no forgiveness.

- Clearly, the cost can be quite high — especially in the erosion of *life quality*.

8) The trainer traces the Type A behavior pattern back to the belief system that drives it, making the following points:

- Underneath every lifestyle pattern lies a set of beliefs that form it and guide personal choices. These beliefs must be examined and perhaps altered before people can successfully change their styles.

- So also with the work addiction trap, common irrational beliefs that lead to workaholism underlie the stress-producing lifestyle. Before people can alter their style and come to grips with their addiction, they must examine and modify the underlying beliefs that guide their daily decisions.

9) The trainer then distributes copies of the **Workaholic Belief Systems** worksheet and asks participants to complete all questions, marking for special attention those beliefs that are particularly troublesome to them.

10) The trainer asks participants to share relevant comments, observations and examples with the entire group.

11) Participants are asked as a total group to generate a list of strategies for coping with the stress of work addiction and for escaping the trap of workaholism.

If the group does not generate many, the trainer may wish to expand on some of the following concepts before closing the session.

- **Be honest with yourself.** The first step in curing any addiction is an honest self-appraisal. Take a look at yourself. Every person suffers from feelings of insecurity. The Type A pattern for dealing with these feelings is to prove oneself by working harder and faster. Do you need achievements in order to feel worthwhile? What insecurity are you hiding by all your racing around? Can you find other methods for becoming lovable?

- **Evaluate your life.** Answer the question, "If I had only one more month to live, what would I do?" Start doing this *today!* Stop now and make that phone call, write that letter, cry if you need to, forgive someone — whatever you need to do — do it now.

- **Choose your fights carefully.** Don't go all out for every challenge that crosses your path. Make choices on when to fight and when to surrender. Learn to float through meetings. Don't run your engine at a breakneck pace all the time. Idle in neutral when there's no need for speed.

- **Practice being creative when you're forced to wait.** Don't get angry, drum your fingers, or fuss about the delay. Stay relaxed and get in touch with your highest self. Write a letter to a friend, memorize poetry, look for beauty within your vision, or learn something from a conversation you strike up with a stranger. Go places where you're forced to wait — then practice patience.

- **Retrieve your whole personality.** Attend to your personal as well as your professional goals. Re-humanize yourself. Concentrate on being a person first. Renew your interest in people. Study faces and learn to love the asymmetry in them. Learn to dream, play, laugh, fantasize, rekindle your curiosity.

- **Learn to see beauty in the small and the weak.** Don't continue to be seduced by size and power; concentrate on appreciating the small and the weak. Take a vacation in your own community. Let the mentally retarded, the chronically ill, the ugly, the sick or very old teach you about matters of the heart. They will accept you for who you are, but they probably won't be impressed by your achievements.

- **Learn that life is unfinished.** Nothing is ever fully completed. To be finished is to be dead. Tell yourself, "I won't finish everything today — and that's okay!" Practice leaving partially completed work on your desk. Remember, life is a journey, not a destination.

VARIATIONS

■ If time permits, the trainer may divide the participants into groups of four to discuss the beliefs which underlie work addiction *(Step 10)*.

■ The coping ideas in *Step 11* could be duplicated and used as a handout.

■ As an added wrinkle, the trainer may begin this session by instructing all participants to put their watches in their pockets so that they aren't able to see what time it is. This will drive the time-pressured workaholics wild. Those who won't comply convict themselves of addiction before they even get into the exercise.

■ For supplementary lecture material on the connection between the "Hurry-up Sickness" and heart disease, the trainer may consult *Type A Behavior and Your Heart* by Friedman and Rosenman, Greenwich: Fawcett Books, 1974.

■ The trainer may want to close with the "Slow Me Down, Lord" prayer from *I Surrender (Stress 1, p 78)* or a rousing chorus of the "Type A Theme Song" from *Singalong 2 (Stress 1, p 125)*.

TRAINER'S NOTES

THE HURRY SICKNESS TEST

You may be addicted to work if you regularly exhibit a number of the following behaviors and attitudes that characterize the Type A pattern. (Check those that apply to you, at least some of the time.)

ENGAGE IN VOCAL EXPLOSIVENESS ____
____ accentuate key words when there's no reason to do so
____ speed up at the end of my sentences

MOVE, WALK, AND EAT RAPIDLY ____

IMPATIENT AT THE RATE OF EVENTS ____
____ hurry speech of others
____ say "yes, yes, uh-huh, yes"
____ finish sentences for others
____ irritated at slow car ahead
____ hate to wait in line or for an appointment
____ "take over" when I can do it faster/better than others
____ irritated with repetitious duties
____ hurry my reading (or read mostly summaries)

POLYPHASIC THOUGHT OR PERFORMANCE ____
____ think or do more than one thing simultaneously — while listening think of tasks, while golfing think of work, while eating read, talk, plan

SELF-ENGROSSED ____
____ bring theme of conversation around to my expertise and interests
____ if not, stay quiet and think about my interests

FEEL VAGUELY GUILTY WHEN RELAXING ____
____ seldom "do nothing" for a few hours (or days)

MISS THE INTERESTING AND LOVELY IN MY PATH ____
____ don't hear birds, see flowers, etc
____ can't remember decorations in a room or office

PREOCCUPIED WITH THINGS *WORTH HAVING* **OR** *WORTH DOING* ____
____ little time for things worth BEING
____ lost the poetic part of me

CHRONIC SENSE OF TIME URGENCY ____
____ schedule more and more in less and less time
____ make few allowances for unforeseen contingencies
____ pride in working best "under pressure"

FEEL COMPETITIVE RELATING TO ANOTHER TYPE A PERSON ____
____ rather than feel compassion for her "illness", I feel challenged to compete and not let her "win"
____ feel hostile or aggressive more quickly with Type A than with Type B people

©1983 Whole Person Press PO Box 3151 Duluth MN 55812   (218) 728-6807

HABITUAL PATTERN OF GESTURES AND/OR NERVOUS TICS _____
___ gestures in conversation (eg, clenched fist, waving finger, table-pounding, etc)
___ spasmodically tighten corners of mouth, clench jaw, constant smile, constant nod of head, etc

BELIEVE SUCCESS IS RELATED TO DOING THINGS FASTER THAN OTHERS ____
___ afraid to slow down
___ feel "unsupported" when I slow down

TRANSLATE LIFE INTO "NUMBERS GAME" _____
___ increasingly evaluate self and work in terms of numbers
___ compare my numbers with the numbers of others

BELIEVE I AM ADDICTED, BUT ALSO BELIEVE THAT I (ALONE?) CAN "GET AWAY WITH IT" AND IT WON'T HURT ME _____

THE TYPE B PROFILE

You're *Type B* (not addicted to work) if you:

1) Are free from *Type A* habits and exhibit none of the traits of work addiction.

2) Accept delays and let others do things at their own pace, without impatience.

3) Enjoy other people and let other people help you.

4) Harbor no free-gloating hostility and feel little need to display or discuss your achievements unless it is demanded by the situation.

5) Play for pleasure and relaxation; enjoy games and sports just for fun — not to compete and to exhibit your superiority.

6) Can relax without guilt.

7) Can work without agitation.

8) Find it easy to allow some tasks to remain uncompleted while you relax and enjoy yourself.

TYPE A OR TYPE B?

Most of us exhibit Type A addictive behavior in some situations and Type B non-addictive behavior in other situations. A "moderately afflicted" Type A workaholic can still turn his "hurry-up sickness" off and on at will.

Type A behavior is a habit, and like any habit it can become addicting. In the early stages of the illness you can still control it; in the latter stages you no longer have control; the illness runs rampant.

The first step in getting a handle on any unhealthy addiction is to make a good, honest self-appraisal. But beware — one characteristic of the Type A workaholic is that she can no longer recognize the addiction in herself!

On the scale below rate yourself and your present behavior. Place an "X" on the continuum.

100% Type A   *100% Type B*
Workaholic   Non-addicted

100/0	90/10	75/25	60/40	50/50	40/60	25/75	10/90	0/100
A B	A B	A B	A B	A B	A B	A B	A B	A B

Factors in my behavior which pushed my rating more toward *Type A:*	Factors in my behavior which pushed my rating more toward *Type B:*

WORKAHOLIC BELIEF SYSTEMS

The four syndromes listed below are typical patterns for workaholics. Do you recognize yourself in the unspoken assumptions and beliefs that undergird the syndromes? As you reflect on your behavior patterns, which of the self-messages motivate you?

The "super" syndrome

___ *"I must always be competent"*
___ *"I must get everything done on time"*
___ *"I don't have the limits of normal people"*

The "workaholic" syndrome

___ *"I must work hard all the time"*
___ *"I must finish work before I play"*
___ *"I must work harder than others"*
___ *"I'm worth more when I work — when I accomplish something I feel more worthwhile"*

The "striving" syndrome

___ *"I must always keep striving to improve myself in every way"*
___ *"No matter how capable I am I could have done better"*

The "tough" syndrome

___ *"Challenges bring out the best in me"*
___ *"I don't need much sleep"*
___ *"I can tolerate pain (I've learned to play even when hurt)"*
___ *"Big boys don't cry"*

In what ways do these beliefs lead me into behaviors that may cause me stress-related health problems?

Observations and comments:

TRAINER'S NOTES

MANAGEMENT STRATEGIES

12 THE AAAbc's OF STRESS MANAGEMENT (p 49)

This coping practicuum teaches a simple paradigm for dealing with stress. Participants practice applying these strategies in role-play situations first and then apply the model to one of their own stressors. (45-60 minutes)

13 PROFESSIONAL SELF-CARE (p 56)

In this two-part exercise participants first assess their personal and professional coping resources, then create a plan for minimizing stress in their work environment. The first part of the exercise makes a wonderful icebreaker. (60 minutes)

14 COPING SKILLS ASSESSMENT (p 63)

In this personal assessment process, participants explore their general coping skills and check out their skill level and usage pattern for 21 different coping techniques. (45-60 minutes)

15 SKILL SKITS (p 68)

This energizing and entertaining exercise fosters participants' creativity and "esprit de corps" while graphically illustrating the wide variety of coping alternatives available to all. (60 minutes)

16 STRESS BUFFER SHIELD (p 71)

Participants develop a personal stress buffer by affirming the qualities, life experiences and coping skills that strengthen and protect them from negative stress. This process is especially effective as an icebreaker or closing affirmation. (20-30 minutes)

12 THE AAAbc's OF STRESS

This coping practicuum teaches a simple paradigm for dealing with stress. Participants practice applying these strategies in role play situations first and then apply the model to one of their own stressors.

GOALS

To explore alternatives for coping with stress.

To practice applying a coping model in hypothetical stressful situations.

To choose an effective stress management strategy for dealing with a specific personal stressor.

GROUP SIZE

Any size

TIME FRAME

45–60 minutes

MATERIALS NEEDED

Blackboard or flipchart; **Stress Scenarios; AAAbc Application Forms**

PROCESS

1) The trainer introduces the *AAAbc* decision-making model for stress management using plenty of examples as he expands on the following points:

- **Stress management is a decision-making process.** When we are feeling the effects of a stressful life position or a stressful lifestyle, we have three major ways we could deal with that stress:
  * <u>A</u>lter it
  * <u>A</u>void it or
  * <u>A</u>ccept it by
    <u>b</u>uilding our resistance or
    <u>c</u>hanging our perception

● All three of these approaches can be effective coping techniques. The trick is choosing the proper approach for the situation at hand and the person involved.

● The first A of the *AAAbc* stands for *Alter* which implies *removing the source of stress* by changing something. Problem-solving, direct communication, organizing, planning and time management are common techniques for altering stress.

☞ *The trainer should illustrate each concept with several examples that vividly demonstrate the strategy (eg, someone who has been saddled with all the arrangements for the ice cream social could alter that stress with good planning and time management or a clear request for help).*

● The second A of the *AAAbc* model stands for *Avoid* which implies *removing oneself from the stressful situation* or figuring out how not to get there in the first place! To conserve stress energy, people sometimes need to walk away, let go, say "no", delegate, withdraw and know their limits so they can "live to fight another day."

☞ *The ice cream social director could avoid the stress by recognizing her limits and resigning from the position or delegating the responsibility.*

● The third A in the AAAbc model stands for *Accept* which involves *equipping oneself physically and mentally for stress*. The b and c of the *AAAbc* model represent this physical and mental preparation.

● b stands for *building resistance*. People can increase their capacity to tolerate stress *physically* through proper diet, regular aerobic exercise and systematic relaxation techniques. Relaxation and exercise provide the double bonus of releasing stored up tension as well! *Mental* resistance is bolstered through positive affirmation, taking time for mental health, and getting clear about goals/values/priorities. *Social* resistance is strengthened by building and maintaining support systems, investing in relationships, clear communication and intimacy. *Spiritual* resistance is especially important in times of high stress. Meditation, prayer, worship, faith and commitment strengthen people.

● c stands for *change*. One way to Accept stress is to *change the way you perceive the situation* or yourself. Changing unrealistic expectations and irrational beliefs such as *"I should succeed at everything I try,"* or *"It would be awful if my spouse were angry with me,"* is a good start. *Building self-esteem and cultivating a positive attitude help as well.* **Redefining the situation in a less stress-provoking way is always an option** — when people play "ain't it funny" or "ain't it grand" instead of "ain't it awful," their stress resistance increases.

2) The trainer models the stress management decision-making process using the *AAAbc* paradigm. He reads one of the **Stress Scenarios** or gives an example of his own to the group.

The trainer asks participants to suggest possible coping options for the stressful situation. As people make their recommendations, the trainer classifies them according to the *AAAbc* model.

After 8–10 ideas have been categorized the group votes on the most effective coping strategy for the situation.

   ☞ *If no one strategy emerges as a clear winner, use this opportunity to illustrate the principle of individual differences — in the same situation different people will have different needs and different responses. The important issue is knowing what works best for you!*

3) Participants divide into groups of six to practice applying the *AAAbc* model to specific stressful situations. The trainer distributes one copy of the **Stress Scenarios** to each group along with enough **AAAbc Application Forms** so that each group has one for each of their scenarios.

4) The trainer instructs the groups to read one scenario out loud and then to brainstorm together a list of management strategies which might work in this situation. One person acts as recorder, summarizing the scene briefly at the top of the **Application Form** and noting all suggestions under their proper categories. If the group gets stuck or off-track, the recorder can ask one of the specific questions posed on the **Application Form.** (5 minutes)

   ☞ *The trainer may want to circulate through the room to "listen in" on the process and act as consultant where needed to clarify the task.*

5) The trainer calls time and asks the group to choose *one* of the suggested strategies as the *Best Option* and record it on the bottom of the **Application Form**. (1 minute)

6) The trainer collects the first round of **Application Forms**. The groups choose another scenario and repeat the process of *Steps 4 and 5*.

   The trainer directs participants to repeat these steps, each time with a different scenario, until the energy level of the group begins to sag. (4 or 5 scenarios are usually plenty!)

7) The trainer reconvenes the group and asks for insights/observations/comments.

   After a few people have shared their experience, the trainer reviews each scenario and reads the *Best Option* solution suggested by each of the groups and again solicits comments from participants.

8) The trainer asks participants to apply the model to their own life situation. He distributes a copy of the **AAAbc Application Form** to everyone and asks them to write a brief scenario of one of their current life stressors. Then they are to answer the questions, brainstorming mentally their own list of coping options. Finally they are to choose one *Best Option* to use in dealing with this stress.

VARIATIONS

- The trainer may want to devise stress scenarios that are especially appropriate to the training group or learning situation. Most of the vignettes in *The Discriminating Feeler (Wellness 1, p 74)* could easily be expanded into stress scenarios.

- In *Step 3* the trainer may want to type the scenarios on note cards and distribute them one at a time for each round of brainstorming. The trainer could choose two or three to give to all the groups, or ask each group to work on a different stress situation.

The chalktalk is based on ideas presented by Joe E Dunlap and J Douglas Stewart in **Keeping the Fire Alive**, *Tulsa: Penwell, 1983.*

AAAbc APPLICATION FORM

SCENARIO

ALTER: *How could you remove the source of stress?*

AVOID: H*ow could you get away from or prevent the stress?*

ACCEPT: *How could you live with the stress?*

Build up your resistance?

Change yourself or your perceptions?

BEST OPTION:

STRESS SCENARIOS

Scenario 1

You are a working parent. You have a long commute and a job that often stretches beyond the boundaries of an eight hour day. You're beat by the time you get home at night and often feel overwhelmed by the dependency needs of others that have to be met before bedtime. You often fall into bed soon after the kids go to sleep so that you can be up by 5:00 am. Lately you've been experiencing physical symptoms that indicate the stress of your lifestyle is getting to you. What could you do?

Scenario 2

You are in your twenties and have just moved to the city to take a new job. You don't know anyone in town except for a couple of people at work. The loneliness is starting to get to you, but you're not the kind of person who does well in the singles bar scene. So you've been spending all your evenings in your apartment reading or watching TV. You're getting more and more depressed. What could you do?

Scenario 3

You have a new supervisor at work who doesn't seem to like you. No matter what you do she is always critical of your efforts. You're beginning to think you'll never be able to please her. What could you do?

Scenario 4

You have a decent job and a reasonable salary but in the current economic climate it's getting harder and harder to make ends meet. Every month is a struggle. You had planned to take a vacation trip this summer but you've decided you'll have to cancel those plans even though your spouse is really counting on going. Now's the time to let your spouse know. What could you do?

Scenario 5

You represent your organization on a community-wide committee that is trying to plan an integrated approach to dealing with pregnant teenagers. You've been meeting twice a month for almost a year without accomplishing much of anything — partly because of politics, partly because of inept leadership. You believe in the purpose of the committee but find yourself tense and irritable after every meeting. It's so frustrating you can hardly stand to go any more. Your supervisor has been raising questions about all the time you've been spending on the project. What should you do?

Scenario 6

Your job takes you away from home several times a month. You've noticed that the first night you're home again after an absence you and your spouse often argue or act in hurtful ways to one another. You are starting to dread coming home after a trip. What could you do?

Scenario 7

You have two children in high school. They are basically good kids and helpful around the house, but recently the older one has been neglecting chores and mercilessly bugging the younger one. Tonight it was complaints about dinner, an argument about whose turn for dishes and slamming doors when you mentioned homework. You feel wound up and ready to snap if you observe one more act of rebellion. What could you do?

13 PROFESSIONAL SELF-CARE

In this two-part exercise participants first assess their personal and professional coping resources, then create a plan for minimizing stress in their work environment. The first part of the exercise makes a wonderful icebreaker.

GOALS

To reduce professionals' resistance to self-care strategies for dealing with stress.

To help participants identify personal resources for stress management.

To explore the possible components of a work environment that maximizes energizers and minimizes stress exhaustion.

GROUP SIZE

Unlimited

TIME FRAME

60 minutes

MATERIALS NEEDED

Blackboard or flipchart; a copy of the **Professional Self-Care Inventory** for each participant.

PROCESS

1) The trainer distributes the **Professional Self-Care Inventory** to participants and asks them to write the name of their profession or work role in the appropriate spaces (eg, nurse, counselor, businessman, saleswoman, supervisor, domestic engineer, etc). She instructs participants to identify their *professional* (Box #1) and *personal* (Box #2) assets on the worksheets. (5 minutes)

   ☞ *If this exercise is used as an icebreaker in a large group, hand out the worksheet as soon as most people are in the room waiting to start. This gets participants involved immediately and reduces the irritation level of*

©1983 Whole Person Press PO Box 3151 Duluth MN 55812   (218) 728-6807

professionals who don't like waiting for stragglers. Write the instructions on the board for latecomers.

2) As soon as most people have finished *Step 1* the trainer explains the importance of positive images in preparing people to tackle difficult issues. She points out that all too often people ignore the rewards of their professions. Yet each item on their asset list is an energy-giver that can be used in preparing them for dealing with the exhaustion of their work role — if they will only activate it as a positive image.

3) The trainer asks participants to share with the whole group a few of the special joyful aspects of their **profession or work role** that they listed in Box #1.

   ☞ *This discussion is limited to professional assets. Personal assets (Box #2) are incorporated in Step 9.*

   In a mixed group, participants should state their work role first and then share their professional assets. Be sure to compliment each person for whatever they share. There are no right and wrong answers.

4) The trainer comments on the list generated by the group, noting the types of rewards participants have identified, summarizing the general tone and affirming the rich assets of the group. She may also want to solicit from the group ideas about how each of these assets might be an on-the-job stress-reducer or stress-preventer.

5) The trainer next asks participants to reflect on a much easier question to answer — "What are the *exhausters* in your *professional* life?" She invites them to use Box #3 for listing all the people, situations, demands, etc of their professional life that drain them, annoy them, distress them, etc. Participants write down their *exhausters*. (2–3 minutes)

   ☞ *The trainer may want to reassure participants that they will not have to disclose any of this information to others in the group. If people seem inhibited or highly concerned, suggest they use a code or symbols.*

6) The trainer directs participants to focus on their *personal* lives and jot down some of the *exhausters* they encounter off-the-job. Participants list these personal drainers, irritators, stressors in Box #4. The trainer encourages people to be as specific and comprehensive as possible in drawing up their lists. (2–3 minutes)

7) The trainer comments that these *exhausters*, both professional and personal, are often the source of much stress and unhappiness for people. She indicates that the remainder of the exercise will be focused on developing a strategy for creating an environment that minimizes exhausters and maximizes energizers.

8) Participants next record the *energizers* in the *professional* (Box #5) and *personal* (Box #6) arenas. They list all the people, situations, things that excite, stimulate, calm, reinforce, or motivate them at work and away from work. (5–6 minutes)

9) The trainer suggests that these energizers provide natural stress buffers. A positive professional self-care plan will probably focus on maximizing these interactions with the environment.

10) The trainer asks participants to review the contents of Boxes #1, #2, #5 and #6 and then brainstorm individually a list of the kinds of work activities that could potentially utilize their assets/energizers alone or in combination. People are to fantasize as many ways as they can imagine to take advantage of their natural gifts and inclinations in a work setting (not necessarily their present job). (5–10 minutes)

☞ *The trainer will need to encourage participants to put on their creative thinking caps and suspend their judgment, writing down all the wild and crazy combinations that occur to them. The point here is to free people up to view themselves as potentially able to create a less stress-producing work environment. Give them some fun and funny examples of your own.*

11) Participants divide into small groups (4–6 people). Each person, in turn, shares his assets/energizers and reads his "work fantasy" list. The group brainstorms even more options to add to the list of potentially enhancing work activities. (20 minutes)

12) After receiving this additional input, each participant evaluates his final list carefully and decides what specific job performance, environment, people relations and role characteristics would be most appropriate for him — for his pace, his time sense, his coping style. The trainer invites each person to write a job description of the "perfect" work situation, given his individual style.

13) The trainer challenges participants to formulate a plan for transforming their current work environments into something that more closely resembles their dream situation. Each person lists at least five steps he could take toward his goal, and chooses one he will try this week.

14) The trainer invites participants to share their transformation plans with the group at large and then closes with a reminder that they should reward themselves for every step they take on the road to more responsible self-care in the workplace. The process is more important than the specific outcome!

VARIATIONS

■ This exercise works especially well for homogeneous professional or paraprofessional groups such as all nurses or all clergy or all managers or all attorneys or all secretaries or all teachers. In this situation, the trainer may want to tailor the worksheet by filling in the name of the profession in advance.

The group could spend more time in *Step 3* exploring the rewards of their profession. As part of *Step 6* the trainer may want to solicit examples of professional exhausters from the group, then do the same for professional energizers in *Step 8*.

■ The trainer may use the first part of this exercise (*Steps 1 and 2*) alone as an icebreaker preceding some other stress assessment or skill development process. Participants pair up or form small groups to discuss professional assets.

■ In an ongoing stress management group, the trainer may want to assign part of this exercise as homework. Participants could share the contents of their "personal" boxes with their spouse and ask for additional feedback about their assets, exhausters and energizers.

Participants could complete *Step 11* (consultation groups) on their own, asking three or more personal or professional friends to brainstorm a list of creative work environments with them.

Submitted by John-Henry Pfifferling.

PROFESSIONAL SELF-CARE INVENTORY

PROFESSIONAL

(1) PROFESSIONAL ASSETS

Make a list of your professional assets. What are the unique, special, rewarding things that are connected with your work/professional role as a _____?

1)   2)

3)   4)

5)   6)

7)   8)

9)   10)

PERSONAL

(2) PERSONAL ASSETS

Make a list of your personal assets. What are your strengths and unique qualities as a person separate from your work/professional role as a _____?

1)   2)

3)   4)

5)   6)

7)   8)

9)   10)

©1983 Whole Person Press PO Box 3151 Duluth MN 55812   (218) 728-6807

PROFESSIONAL SELF-CARE INVENTORY

(3)	(5)	
		PROFESSIONAL
(4)	(6)	
		PERSONAL

TRAINER'S NOTES

14 COPING SKILLS ASSESSMENT

In this personal assessment process, participants explore their general coping skills and check out their skill level and usage pattern for 21 different coping techniques.

GOALS

To assess and affirm stress management skills participants already use well.

To expand personal repertoire of coping skills.

To identify target skills for future development.

GROUP SIZE

Unlimited; could be adapted for use with individuals.

TIME FRAME

45–60 minutes

MATERIALS NEEDED

Skills Assessment worksheets for all participants.

PROCESS

1) The trainer introduces the concept of stress management as a learned skill and suggests that we all have a personal repertoire of coping skills that we have developed over the years. We can always learn more skills, too! Since no skill works every time, the more coping options we have the more likely we will deal successfully with the stress we encounter.

2) The trainer highlights the four basic stress management strategies to be considered here, giving several examples for each.
   - **Personal Management Skills:**
       Organizing your time/energy expenditure.
   - **Relationship Skills:**
       Changing your interactions with the environment.
   - **Outlook Skills:**
       Mind-changing techniques for controlling your attitude.
   - **Self-Care Skills:**
       Building your strength, stamina, and outlets for tension.

©1983 Whole Person Press PO Box 3151 Duluth MN 55812 (218) 728-6807

3) The trainer asks participants to reflect on their own stress skill patterns and identify which strategy they are most likely to use when they are under pressure.

4) The trainer then asks for a show of hands.

✔ How many people chose personal management skills as their area of strength?

✔ Relationship skills? Outlook skills? Self-care skills?

The trainer comments on the diversity/similarity in the group.

5) Participants next identify their weakest coping strategy area — the general approach that they are least likely to use in combating stress.

6) Again the trainer asks the group to vote, this time indicating their weakest strategies. The trainer comments on the overall pattern in the group.

7) The trainer distributes the **Skills Assessment** worksheet and points out that knowing how to use a stress skill and actually using it are two different issues. A person can be highly skilled in a specific coping technique and never use it. It's also possible to use a technique frequently and ineptly.

Participants are asked to rate themselves on their skill level and usage as the trainer describes each skill individually in detail.

☞ *This could turn into a long, boring process unless the trainer spices things up. One of the best ways to keep the energy level high is to involve participants in experimenting briefly with some of the skills. Several group energizers in this volume could be used to illustrate skills (I Surrender!, 5–4–3–2–1 Contact, Stretch, Humorous Interludes, etc). Or brainstorm your own list of creative quickies.*

8) The trainer invites participants to summarize their present stress skill pattern by answering the first four questions on the bottom of the worksheet.

9) The trainer then asks everyone to look toward the future and imagine what skills they might want to be using six months or a year from now. Participants answer the last four questions identifying target skills for further development as well as skills to maintain or let go for now.

10) The trainer asks for questions/insights/comments from the group and uses these to summarize the session content.

VARIATIONS

■ *Skill Skits, Stress 1, p 68*, is an excellent follow-up to this exercise.

■ Before *Step 11*, participants could divide into dyads or small groups to share their stress skills profiles and resolutions for change.

TRAINER'S NOTES

Adapted from the STRESS SKILLS Participant Workbook, Duluth MN: Whole Person Associates, 1979.

STRESS SKILLS ASSESSMENT

	SKILL LEVEL				SKILL USE			
	unskilled	semi-skilled	proficient	expert	never	rarely	occasionally	regularly
PERSONAL MANAGEMENT SKILLS *organizing your time/energy expenditure*								
VALUING: *investing self correctly*								
PLANNING: *moving toward goals*								
COMMITMENT: *saying "yes"*								
TIME USE: *setting priorities*								
PACING: *controlling the tempo*								
RELATIONSHIP SKILLS *interacting with your environment*								
CONTACT: *reaching out to others*								
LISTENING: *tuning in to others*								
ASSERTIVENESS: *saying "no"*								
FIGHT: *standing your ground*								
FLIGHT: *leaving the scene*								
NEST-BUILDING: *creating a "home"*								
OUTLOOK SKILLS *changing your mind, choosing your attitude*								
RELABELING: *a new perspective*								
SURRENDER: *saying "goodbye"*								
FAITH: *accepting your limits*								
IMAGINATION: *laughing, creating*								
WHISPER: *talking nicely to yourself*								

SELF-CARE SKILLS *building your strength,* *stamina and outlets for tension*	SKILL LEVEL						SKILL USE	
	unskilled	semi-skilled	proficient	expert	never	rarely	occasionally	regularly
EXERCISE: *fine-tuning your body*								
EATING: *feeding your body*								
GENTLENESS: *wearing kid gloves*								
RELAXATION: *letting go of tension*								
STRETCHING: *loosening up*							/	

AT PRESENT:

My best skills (highest skill level)

My underdeveloped skills (lowest skill level)

The skills I use most often (highest use)

My underutilized skills (lowest use)

FOR THE FUTURE:

Skills I've neglected — I'd like to start using them again

Skills I'm no good at now, but I'd like to learn and practice them

Skills I'd like to maintain — I know I'll need them

Skills I'd like to use less —time to put these on the back burner

15 SKILL SKITS

This energizing and entertaining exercise fosters participants' creativity and "esprit de corps" while graphically illustrating the wide variety of coping alternatives available to all.

GOALS

To engage participants in an exploration of a wide variety of coping strategies.

To encourage participants' creativity and high energy involvement in the learning process.

To promote team building within small sharing groups.

GROUP SIZE

This exercise works best with 50–100 persons (allowing for 12–25 small groups of four persons each).

TIME FRAME

60 minutes

MATERIALS NEEDED

Blackboard; a list of coping skills for each participant.

PROCESS

☞ *This exercise assumes that the trainer has her own list of 10–20 stress management strategies to be explored by the group or she may use the Stress Skills Assessment from* **Coping Skills Assessment (Stress 1, p 63).**

1) The trainer introduces the subject of coping and briefly outlines her broad general strategies for coping.

2) The trainer divides participants into small groups of 4–6 persons each, or utilizes previously formed sharing units. Participants are asked to gather in small groups, while staying within voice range of the trainer, so they can receive further instructions.

---

3) The trainer informs participants that she will come around to each group and assign them each a different skill to discuss. The groups are to focus on three questions:

✔ What is the skill? (a definition)

✔ In what stressful situations could it be useful?

✔ How could a person develop expertise in using the skill?

☞ *Write the three questions on the board.*

4) The trainer goes around as rapidly as possible, distributing the coping skills list and assigning each group a different skill.

☞ *If there are more skills than groups, the trainer should pick and assign those most interesting to her, remembering which skills have been left out.*

If there are more groups than skills, tell some groups they are to make up a "mystery skill" that is not on the list, but would be helpful for coping.

5) After groups have had 5–10 minutes to "warm up" to their skill focus, the trainer describes the skit-writing process.

➤ Small groups are to spend 20 minutes designing and rehearsing a 30 second TV commercial that sells the rest of the participants on the value of their skill.

➤ In the skit-writing and performance process, the talents of every member should be used.

➤ Be sure to have fun and be as creative as possible.

☞ *Some people may need reassurance that this is a serious task. The trainer needs to state clearly that in 20 minutes sharp, they will perform their commercial for the rest of the participants. Remind them of the 30 second time limit.*

After 15 minutes, remind participants that they have only 5 minutes until "show time." Encourage them to rehearse their commercial so they are really ready.

6) After the groups have had 20 minutes for planning, the trainer reconvenes the participants and announces that the show will begin. Participants are instructed to listen and learn from the skills that others present.

The trainer directs that the skits will be performed in the order the skills appear on the coping skills list. (This will allow the "on deck" group to get prepared.) All skits are to be performed from the "front" of the room.

The trainer points out that at $100,000/minute . . . groups must move quickly and keep within their 30 second slot or it will cost them dearly!

☞ *The performance of skits will provide maximum humor, energy and insights if the pace moves rapidly. Don't let them drag on. Don't allow long pauses between skits!*

7) One-by-one the trainer calls each group by announcing, "If you've got too much stress you might deal with it by *(the next skill)*." The trainer politely thanks each group following their skit.

☞ *Be sure to hand the microphone to each group, or else many will not be heard! Be prepared to be "roasted" yourself by some groups!*

8) After all skits are completed the trainer asks the groups to give themselves a hand.

9) Small groups meet to discuss the stress they experienced in completing the skill skit tasks, and to identify the numerous skills they used individually and as a group in coping with the "threat" of the task.

10) The trainer reconvenes the entire group and asks for comments/observations/insights on the process.

VARIATIONS

■ The **Skill Skits** may be treated as a contest. At the close of the skits the trainer may award humorous citations of merit to various groups. Or the trainer may appoint a "panel of judges" before the skits are performed. The panel will announce their decisions at the close of the session.

■ The 30 second commercials may be lengthened to 60 seconds if fewer groups are participating, but they should never be longer than 60 seconds, or they will drag.

■ This energizing exercise can be preceded or followed by a more serious individual assessment of personal skill strengths and weaknesses such as *Coping Skills Assessment (Stress 1, p 63).*

16 STRESS BUFFER SHIELD

Participants develop a personal stress buffer by affirming the qualities, life experiences and coping skills that strengthen and protect them from negative stress. This process is especially effective as an icebreaker or closing affirmation.

GOALS
To affirm personal qualities that buffer the effects of stress.

GROUP SIZE
Unlimited; works well with individuals, too.

TIME FRAME
20–30 minutes

MATERIALS NEEDED
Stress Buffer Shield worksheets for all participants.

PROCESS
1) The trainer describes a *stress buffer* as a personal store of constructive coping skills that help people transform stress into a positive force and protects them from breaking down under pressure.

2) The trainer distributes the **Stress Buffer Shields** and invites people to reflect on the qualities that comprise their personal stress buffers. Participants write down these life experiences, support networks, attitudes, self-care habits and action skills in the appropriate section of the shield. (5 minutes)

    ☞ *The trainer may want to describe each shield section in detail and give examples.*

3) Participants pair up with a neighbor or form small groups and share their stress buffer shields with one another. (10–20 min)

4) The trainer reconvenes the group and asks for observations and insights. The trainer uses participants' comments as a springboard to the next learning module or as a summary of stress management concepts.

©1983 Whole Person Press PO Box 3151 Duluth MN 55812   (218) 728-6807

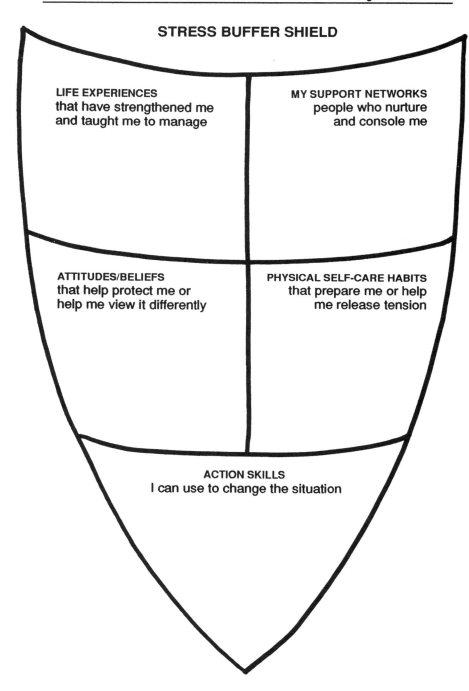

STRESS BUFFER SHIELD

LIFE EXPERIENCES
that have strengthened me
and taught me to manage

MY SUPPORT NETWORKS
people who nurture
and console me

ATTITUDES/BELIEFS
that help protect me or
help me view it differently

PHYSICAL SELF-CARE HABITS
that prepare me or help
me release tension

ACTION SKILLS
I can use to change the situation

SKILL BUILDERS

17 UNWINDING (p 73)
Participants explore the stress-relaxation connection from both the academic and experiential perspectives in this revitalizing skill-builder. (20-30 minutes)

18 I SURRENDER! (p 78)
In three exercises that demonstrate surrender as a coping skill, participants launch a "goodbye" ship, practice the "allowing attitude" and pray for a slower pace.
(2-5 minutes)

19 HUMOROUS INTERLUDES (p 82)
In this coping practicuum collection participants use music, a movie and their imaginations to practice generating the healing power of laughter. (5-10 minutes)

20 5-4-3-2-1 CONTACT (p 86)
In this energizing skill-builder participants experiment with different styles of initiating contact with others. (20-30 minutes)

17 UNWINDING

Participants explore the stress-relaxation connection from both the academic and experiential perspectives in this revitalizing skill-builder.

GOALS

To explore the relationship between stress and relaxation.

To experience a state of profound relaxation.

GROUP SIZE

Unlimited

TIME FRAME

20–30 minutes

MATERIALS NEEDED

Unwinding-Relaxation script; cassette recorder with meditative music (optional).

PROCESS

> ☞ *Breath-Less (Stress 1, p 116) and Tension Hurts (Stress 1, p 133) provide an excellent warm-up to this routine, especially for groups that are resistant to the idea of relaxation.*

1) The trainer introduces the concept of systematic relaxation as the natural antidote to stress.

- The stress response is a marvelous mind/body mechanism that gears us up to meet dangerous situations.

- **Unfortunately, most of us run up the danger flag too often and are left with the residual side effects of chronic stress** — unresolved muscle tension, elevated blood pressure, increased heartbeat and general arousal. Eventually this tension, arousal and tightness begin to seem normal. Chronic tension is bound to breed some long-range consequences such as knotted muscles, headache, joint and spine problems.

- **Systematic relaxation reverses the physiological effects of the emergency stress response** by regulating breathing and reducing unconscious muscular tension. We can't experience both stress and relaxation at the same time. So — if we relax in a potentially stressful situation, we can prevent the stress response. If we've already stressed ourselves, relaxation can reverse the process.

- **Many of our negative coping habits are attempts to induce relaxation** (e.g. cigarettes, alcohol, tranquilizers, eating). Unwinding without chemicals is a much healthier option.

- **Relaxation is a skill we were born with** and unlearned over the years. Anyone can re-learn it. As with learning any skill, the process takes practice and persistence. At first it takes more time, seems awkward, uncomfortable, ineffective. It's tempting to discard the whole idea as "taking too much time" or "being silly."

  Yet with practice the body will relax in seconds — on command — whenever you need to reduce your stress level, to take time out or simply to revitalize yourself.

2) The trainer may want to describe the variety of techniques people use to relax — yoga, exercise, stretching, breathing, meditation, progressive relaxation, autogenics, T'ai chi, visualization, etc. This exercise uses a generic "allowing" process for letting go of tension combined with autogenic suggestions.

3) The trainer invites participants to find a comfortable posture, settle back and prepare to experience a refreshing relaxation break.

   ☞ *The trainer may want to dim the lights and/or turn on some soothing background music such as Pachelbell's Canon in D or a flute solo.*

4) The trainer reads the **Unwinding-Relaxation** script.

   ☞ *Read the script very slowly pausing at the (. . .) markings and stretching out the words. At the end of the script allow plenty of time for people to "return" to the room before turning up the lights or intruding with loud sounds.*

5) The trainer may ask for comments or observations from the group.

UNWINDING-RELAXATION SCRIPT

... This exercise will help you learn the skill of deep relaxation which is so important for stress reduction, stress management and overall health and well-being ... Get comfortable now ... find a relaxed position and allow yourself to concentrate fully on these instructions ...

... Take a deep breath in through your nose ... and as you let it out through your mouth ... allow your eyes to close slowly and comfortably ... Let your body begin to relax and unwind ... Take another deep breath ... and as you exhale let it carry all the tension out of your body ... Allow a feeling of peacefulness to descend over you ... A pleasant and enjoyable sensation of being comfortable and at ease ...

... Now turn your attention to your body and begin to pay close attention to the sensations you experience ... notice the signals your body is sending you ... Find the place in your body that seems most tense ... and allow that muscle to let go of its hold ... Begin to let all your muscles ... all over your body ... give up their hold and go limp ... Now is the time to let go of whatever tension you have been holding on to ... Focus again on your breathing ... filling yourself up as you breathe in ... and letting that tension go when you breathe out ...

... Now direct your attention to the top of your head ... and allow a feeling of relaxation to begin there ... Let that feeling of relaxation spread downward through your body ... Let the small muscles of your scalp relax ... and now allow all the muscles of your forehead to relax and let go ... Pay special attention to your forehead ... let yourself really *feel* the muscle there giving up its hold ... Feel your eyebrows sagging down ... Let all the muscles around the sides and back of your head relax fully and completely ... Imagine that your ears are even drooping under their own weight ... Now allow your cheek and face muscles to relax and let go ... let your jaw muscles relax ... and allow your jaw to drop slightly ... Allow the muscles of your lips and chin to relax and grow limp ... Now all the muscles of your head and face have let go ... and are smooth and relaxed ...

... Next, let the muscles of your neck relax slightly ... tensing them only enough to hold your head upright and balanced easily in position ... Let the feeling of relaxation spread into your throat ... and down the sides of your neck ... into your shoulders ... Allow your shoulders to become heavy and sag downward ... as you relax all your neck and throat and shoulder muscles ...

©1983 Whole Person Press PO Box 3151 Duluth MN 55812   (218) 728-6807

. . . Now, allow the feeling of relaxation you're experiencing to spread downward to the muscles of your chest and upper back . . . Feel the relaxation there as the muscles release their hold . . . Feel the relaxation there . . . Now, let your shoulder muscles go completely limp . . . and allow your arms to rest heavily . . . with your hands in your lap or on your thighs . . . Feel your arms growing very heavy . . . and relax all the muscles of your forearms, hands and fingers . . . Let the tension flow right out your fingertips . . . You are feeling very calm . . . and relaxed . . . and comfortable throughout your upper body . . .

. . . Notice your breathing for a few seconds . . . notice how regular it has become . . . Let that feeling of deep relaxation spread fully through your chest . . . down through the muscles of your back . . . and down into your arms . . . As you do so . . . allow your stomach muscles to relax completely and totally . . . Your stomach will probably sag just a bit as the muscles release their hold . . . Allow that sagging to occur and relax the muscles of your sides . . . the muscles of your shoulder blades . . . and the small of your back . . . Let all the muscles of your spine relax . . . let go all the way from your skull down to the tip of your spine . . . Simply allow all of the muscles of your stomach and sides and back to experience a sensation of warmth . . . and heaviness . . . relaxing more and more deeply . . .

. . . Now, relax the large muscles of your thighs . . . and let them go completely limp . . . feel all your muscles so relaxed that they feel as though they're turning to jelly . . . Your whole body is becoming profoundly relaxed . . . Feel that relaxation now and enjoy it . . . Now, focus on the muscles of your buttocks . . . and let that relaxation spread into the front of your lower legs . . . into your shin muscles . . . into your ankles . . . allowing your ankles to feel free and loose . . . Now, wiggle your toes once or twice . . . and let all of the muscles of your feet give up their hold completely . . . Your whole body is extremely relaxed and comfortable . . .

. . . Simply enjoy these sensations of profound relaxation throughout your body . . . notice that you can feel even more relaxed as you become aware of the warmth in your arms and hands . . . Feel this warmth and allow it to increase . . . Allow your arms to feel extremely heavy and completely limp . . . feel this growing sensation of warmth spreading way out to your fingertips . . . Concentrate closely on your hands and your arms . . . and allow the feeling of pleasant heaviness and warmth to increase by itself . . . Simply observe the process and encourage it . . . Now allow those same feelings of heaviness and warmth to spread throughout your legs . . . Concentrate closely on the sensations in your legs . . . and let them become very, very heavy . . . very heavy and very warm . . . Your arms and legs are so heavy and so warm . . . Your entire body now is profoundly

*relaxed . . . and you feel only a pleasant overall sensation of
heaviness . . . warmth and peace . . .*

*. . . Now, I'd like you to turn your attention to your breathing . . . and
without interfering with your breathing in any way . . . simply observe
it . . . feel the slow, peaceful rise and fall of your stomach as your breath
flows slowly in . . . and slowly out of your body . . . Don't try to hurry your
breathing or slow it down . . . Just notice your breathing . . . and observe its
slow, steady process . . . Imagine that you've just discovered the steady
rising and falling of your stomach . . . and that you're observing it with
curiosity and respect . . . Wait patiently for each breath to arrive . . . and
notice its passing . . . Notice, too, the brief periods of quiet after one breath
passes and before the next one arrives . . . Now, continue to observe this
breathing process and begin to count your breaths as they arrive . . . As the
first one comes, watch it closely and hear yourself mentally say,
"one" . . . Wait patiently for the next one and count, "two" . . . Continue
until you've counted 25 breaths . . . not allowing any other thoughts to
distract you . . .*

> ☞ *The trainer should pause here long enough to count 25 or
> 30 of her own breaths and then gently continue the
> narration, allowing his voice to get progressively stronger
> and more definite.*

*. . . Now you're deeply relaxed . . . and you can return to this peaceful state
whenever you want to . . . Take a few moments now to pay close attention to
this relaxed feeling . . . all over your body . . . and memorize it as carefully
as you can . . . Store the entire feeling of your whole body in your
memory . . . so that later you can retrieve it and relax yourself at will . . .*

*. . . When you feel ready to direct your awareness outside . . . and return to
this place . . . allow yourself all the time you need to wake up your
body . . . and to bring it back to its usual level of alertness and
responsiveness . . . Wiggle your fingers and toes . . . move your arms and
legs a little bit . . . shrug your shoulders . . . turn your head . . . but keep
your eyes closed for a few seconds longer . . . as you experience all parts of
your body reawakening . . . Then, when you are ready, take a nice deep
breath . . . open your eyes . . . and allow your body to feel fully alive and
flowing with plenty of energy.*

18 I SURRENDER!

In three exercises that demonstrate surrender as a coping skill, participants launch a "goodbye" ship, practice the "allowing attitude" and pray for a slower pace.

GOALS

To reinforce the importance of "letting go" as a stress management strategy.

To illustrate the mind-body-spirit connection.

GROUP SIZE

Unlimited

TIME FRAME

2–5 minutes

MATERIALS NEEDED

A blank 8.5" X 11" sheet of paper for each participant

PROCESS

GOODBYE

1) The trainer asks participants to focus on a life problem, big or small, that they wish to get rid of. Participants write a brief description of the problem or life stress in the center of an 8.5" X 11" sheet of paper.

   Next, the trainer asks them to expand their problem statement with phrases and words that accentuate its most negative aspects.

2) The trainer instructs participants to make a paper airplane, using the sheet on which they have described their problem.

3) Participants are then invited to spend two minutes talking to their problem (swearing at it, whispering, saying goodbye, telling it you'll miss it, etc). They then prepare to "kiss it off" with a clean goodbye.

4) On the count of three, participants all simultaneously sail their planes (and problems) away — with a loud group cheer.

5) The trainer asks people to check in with themselves to make sure it was okay to surrender this problem.

☞ *This is a good time to talk about secondary gains. Really challenge participants to consider what it will mean to give up this life stress.*

For all those people who really aren't willing and ready to give up their problem, the trainer suggests they admit it and go retrieve their airplanes — symbolically reclaiming their responsibility for choosing to hold on to their problem for now.

6) The "freed-up" participants are to sound out a total group sigh of relief and relaxation. This sigh is to be repeated three or four times until the volume increases, and shoulders, arms and whole body are engaged in the sigh of relief.

7) The trainer may ask for comments from the group and use these to explore further the issues involved in using surrender as a coping skill.

THE ALLOWING ATTITUDE

☞ *This demonstration takes only a moment and would fit well in a general discussion of mind/body relationships or as part of a presentation on relaxation, autogenics or biofeedback training.*

1) The trainer introduces the concept that thoughts can create physiological changes and invites participants to take part in a brief demonstration.

2) The trainer instructs participants to interlace their fingers (as in praying with folded hands).

Once everyone has achieved the proper position, the trainer asks them to fully extend their index fingers only (palm to palm, pointing upward — as in "here is the church, here is the steeple."

Keeping the other fingers down and the base of the index fingers together, participants next pull back the tips of their index fingers until they are as far separate as possible.

3) The trainer suggests that while they look at the space between their fingers, participants repeat to themselves, "fingers come together."

4) Most people will find that the fingers *do* move together, particularly when they *allow* rather than *prevent* or *force* the response to occur.

☞ *The trainer may point out that this exercise is often used to identify persons who are responsive to "suggestion" and autogenic training. Those people who did not "allow" their fingers to come together may have difficulty "letting go" enough to benefit from such coping techniques.*

5) The trainer asks for insights/observations from the group and uses those comments to underscore the importance of the "allowing attitude" in stress management — especially for those stressors over which we have little or no control.

SLOW ME DOWN LORD

☞ *This exercise is especially effective following a discussion of stress-provoking lifestyle patterns such as Type A Behavior or after an exploration of stress and personal values. (Lifetrap 1, Stress 1, p 37)*

1) The trainer makes a few comments about the importance of slowing down and letting go in dealing with life stress — especially the stress we bring on ourselves by our pace and our unrealistic expectations.

Slow Me Down, Lord

Slow me down, Lord! Ease the pounding of my heart by the quieting of my mind. Steady my hurried pace with the vision of the eternal reach of time. Give me, amidst the confusion of my day, the calmness of the everlasting hills. Break the tensions of my nerves and muscles with the soothing music of the singing streams that live in my memory.

Help me to know the magical, restoring power of sleep. Teach me the art of taking Minute Vacations . . . of slowing down to look at a flower, to chat with a friend, to pat a dog, to read a few lines from a good book, to fish, to dream. Remind me each day of the fable of the hare and the tortoise that I may know that the race is not always to the swift; that there is more in life than increasing speed.

Let me look upward into the branches of the towering oak and know that it grew great and strong because it grew slowly and well. Slow me down, Lord, and inspire me to send my roots deep into the soil of life's enduring values that I may grow upward toward the stars of my greater destiny.

TRAINER'S NOTES

The Allowing Attitude, a traditional T' ai chi exercise, was submitted by David X Swenson. Slow Me Down, Lord was submitted by Mary O' Brien Sippel who learned it from a Stress Skills seminar participant. The author is unknown.

19 HUMOROUS INTERLUDES

In this coping practicuum collection participants use music, a movie and their imaginations to practice generating the healing power of laughter.

GOALS
To explore laughter as a coping skill.

To experience laughter as a tension reducer.

GROUP SIZE
Unlimited

TIME FRAME
5–10 minutes

MATERIALS NEEDED
Beloved Husband of Irma: film

Flight of Fancy: A Walk in the Rain

PROCESS

THE BEST MEDICINE

1) The trainer introduces the concept of laughter as "the best medicine" for stress, touching on some or all of the following points:

- **Laughter is healthy**. Norman Cousins documented his successful experience with laughter therapy as a remedy for degenerative spinal disease in **Anatomy of an Illness** (W W Norton, 1980).

- **Laughter is a natural tension reducer**. Dr William Fry from Stanford University describes laughter as a form of internal jogging. Muscles tense as we wait for the punch line or the ultimate incongruity. Then at the point our giggles erupt, the muscles of the face, neck, chest, belly and diaphragm all get a good work-out. Laughter stimulates the cardiovascular system and exercises the lungs.

©1983 Whole Person Press PO Box 3151 Duluth MN 55812   (218) 728-6807

As the laughter subsides, the muscles all relax profoundly until the tension level falls substantially below the pre-laugh level. Relaxation benefits may last up to 45 minutes. In general, the more intense the laughter, the more relaxing and the longer the effect.

- **Laughter is a natural pain-reliever.** Laughter helps control pain by distracting our attention from the pain, by reducing tension that may be contributing to the pain, by changing our perspective or expectations, and by actually creating physiological changes that reduce pain. Recent research indicates that laughter stimulates the production of endorphins — our body's own natural pain-killers. Hysteria or hilarity are not necessary — delight, mirth and amusement trigger the reaction too!

- **Humor relieves stress by** allowing us to perceive the paradoxes of life from an emotional distance. In laughing and joking about a life situation, we can separate ourselves from an annoying or uncomfortable incident and reduce our consequent stress level. Laughter is especially helpful for those times when our stress is of our own making — or totally beyond our control.

- **People like to be around others with a good sense of humor.**

2) The trainer points out that we often underutilize this healthy coping resource because we're afraid to "look silly". He challenges participants to experiment together with generating healthy laughter.

3) The trainer asks everyone to stand and join in singing a song together (something peppy like "Humoresque" or "Deck the Halls" work well). Instead of singing the words, everyone sings "ha-ha-ha-ha-ha-ha" until they're rolling on the floor! A second and third tune are solicited from the group.

   ☞ *The trainer's attitude and willingness to appear foolish here will make or break the exercise. Encourage people to exaggerate and enjoy the process. Some groups respond to the challenge of "keeping a straight face" during the songs.*

4) The trainer asks those who feel more relaxed as a result of the laughter break to raise their hands and describe their experience, if they care to.

5) The trainer solicits comments from the group on the use of laughter as a stress management skill. Participants may suggest specific situations where humor would be an appropriate stress reducer, or give personal examples of beneficial laughter from their life.

VARIATION

■ With an adventurous group, the trainer could suggest a game of "Minne-ha-ha." Everyone lies in a line on the floor, each person with her head lying on the next person's tummy. The first person in line says very loudly, "Minne-ha-ha-ha", the next, "Minne-ha-ha-ha-ha," and so on, adding a "ha" for each new person until everyone's in stitches.

BELOVED HUSBAND OF IRMA

☞ *This entertaining movie needs no introduction or discussion. It works best just before a break, after people have been sitting still for awhile.*

1) The trainer invites participants to join in a tension-reducing laughter break.

2) The movie **Beloved Husband of Irma** is shown to the group.

☞ *This hilarious 7-minute film of a stressful scene from the stall of a men's room usually brings down the house. Only the most pristine would be offended at the humor. Available from: MTI Teleprograms Inc, 3710 Commercial Ave, Northbrook IL 60062 1-800-323-5343. Purchase: $195.00. Rental: $50.00*

FLIGHT OF FANCY

1) The trainer points out that humor and creativity share a common root — the ability to recognize and appreciate the incongruities of life. Both of these coping strategies depend on a lively imagination that can be exercised and enhanced with practice.

2) The trainer invites participants to join in an imagination laughter break using the **A Walk in the Rain** script.

☞ *Invite people to shut their eyes if they wish — some people visualize better that way. Read the script slowly allowing plenty of time to get each image clearly in mind before moving on to the next.*

A WALK IN THE RAIN

Picture a man walking in a rainstorm. It's pouring. He is wearing a new, three piece suit and marching with dignity down the street, an umbrella over his head. But the umbrella has no cloth or plastic. It's just a skeleton of spokes. Give him a red tie that's bleeding all over his white shirt. Now give him short pants, white socks and cowboy boots. Have him meet someone. What do they say?

3) Participants pair up with a partner and recount their visualizations, embellishing the story with vivid details and making the description as funny as possible. (5 minutes)

VARIATIONS

■ The trainer could make up absurd visualizations involving the people in the group or their profession or work setting.

■ After *Step 3* participants could make up a visualization for their partners and guide them through the imaging process. After 2–3 minutes the pair would switch roles.

TRAINER'S NOTES

20 5-4-3-2-1 CONTACT

In this energizing skill-builder participants experiment with different styles of initiating contact with others.

GOALS

To highlight the importance of interpersonal relationships as a stress management strategy.

To experiment with different forms of making contact.

GROUP SIZE

Works best with 20 or more people; adaptable to smaller groups.

TIME FRAME

20–30 minutes

MATERIALS NEEDED

Participants need blank paper for making notes.

PROCESS

1) The trainer announces that this will be an experimental exploration of contact as a stress management skill.

2) The trainer invites participants to stand up and move about the room. During the next five minutes they are to make contact in whatever way they wish with five other persons in the group.

   ☞ *This instruction may get a few laughs and probably many puzzled looks. The trainer should encourage people to go ahead and use their natural style to make contact with five individuals — do whatever is normal and comfortable for them.*

3) After five minutes, the trainer calls time and reconvenes the group. She asks participants to jot some notes to themselves about their contacting style. The following questions should help people uncover their patterns:

   ✔ What did you notice about your contacts?

   ✔ Did you initiate contact? Or were you holding back, hoping others would come to you?

✔ Did you touch any of your contacts? How did you decide?

✔ How about eye contact?

✔ Who talked, who listened?

✔ How was your style here similar to/different from your "usual" style of making contact?

4) The trainer asks for comments from the group and gives feedback on how she observed the group interacting.

5) The trainer may want to expand on the following issues if they do not come up spontaneously in the dialogue:

● **Human beings need contact with other human beings.** Contact energizes people and is a powerful stress reliever. Unfortunately we often shut ourselves off from the contact we need.

● **We frequently hold ourselves back** from the support and other goodies we might get from people because we don't want to appear ridiculous or intrusive.

● Often we have strong urges to reach out to others but keep the lid on because the intensity of our feelings scares us or we fear the possible sexual overtones.

● Sometimes we can't make contact just because we feel awkward or embarrassed or uncertain or unworthy.

● **Contact skills are learned behaviors** — we all can practice making contact in new ways, with new people, with new attitudes. The reward is likely to be an ever-expanding support network that energizes and nurtures us.

☞ *The trainer may want to insert some more specific information on assertiveness or communication skills as part of this chalktalk.*

6) The trainer points out that this group is a good, safe place to experiment with building contact skills. She suggests that during the contacting acting exercise every person was undoubtedly cautious about how they reached out and hesitant to act on some of their urges.

7) The trainer invites participants to try the contacting exercise again. They are again to make contact with five different individuals, but this time they are to do so in a way that breaks their normal rules for reaching out, that stretches their personal boundaries. Participants are to act on their urges, and to follow different urges with different people.

8) The trainer calls time after five minutes and directs people to reflect on the second round of contacts:

✔ What was your energy level compared to the first round?

✔ When did you feel most alive?

✔ What was most inhibiting?

✔ In which contact did you feel most free?

✔ What was your favorite interaction?

✔ How would this contact skill help you deal with one of your stressors?

9) The trainer requests insights/observations from the group and uses them to summarize and reinforce the major concepts.

VARIATIONS

■ As part of *Step 7* participants could re-contact the same five people, as in Round 1, but with a different style. After each contact the partners could compare notes on how they felt about the interactions in both rounds.

TRAINER'S NOTES

Submitted by Mary O'Brien Sippel

ACTION PLANNING

21 GETTING OUT OF MY BOX (p 89)
In this reflective exercise participants examine the chronically stressful situations in their lives and explore ways of caring for themselves in spite of the painful life circumstances that may limit them. (60-90 minutes)

22 ONE STEP AT A TIME (p 102)
This nine-part guide leads participants step-by-step through a creative planning process for coping with a stress-related problem. (20-30 minutes)

23 POSTSCRIPT (p 108)
In this action planning exercise participants write themselves letters which are then collected by the trainer and mailed sometime later as a reminder of the learning that took place. (15 minutes)

24 COPING SKILL AFFIRMATION (p 110)
This exercise is designed to affirm participants' positive stress management coping skills, and is most effective at the conclusion of an ongoing learning experience. (60 minutes)

21 GETTING OUT OF MY BOX

In this reflective exercise participants examine the chronically stressful situations in their lives and explore ways of caring for themselves in spite of the painful life circumstances that may limit them.

GOALS

To help participants recognize and label the sources of chronic distress in their lives.

To help participants make intentional choices in deciding what to do about the situations that "box them in."

To allow participants the experience of being lovable and acceptable in spite of their personal limitations and chronic stressors.

TIME FRAME

60–90 minutes

GROUP SIZE

Any size; also adaptable for use with individuals.

MATERIALS NEEDED

My Personal Box worksheet for each participant.

PROCESS

☞ *This exercise is particularly effective for people who find themselves in one of two kinds of circumstances: (1) they are surrounded by some major life problems that they cannot change; or (2) they have tried to alter their lifestyle but have repeatedly been "unsuccessful."*

A. WARM UP (5 minutes)

1) The trainer introduces the concepts of personal limitations and chronic stress, connecting these themes to the goals of the exercise.

- All people are "boxed in" by some things that limit them — that cause them chronic distress.

- The source of these boxes can be internal or external, physical, mental, spiritual or social.

- Some of the most common "boxes" people experience include:
  Expectations and beliefs: the "I shoulds" of life.
  Habits: overeating, smoking, drinking.
  People: restricted relationships, illness, chronic disappointment.
  Employment issues: unemployment, financial pressures, rules, expectations.
  Personal failures.
  Personal limitations.
  Diseases.

- We call these boxes "chronic" stressors because that's what they are. They are stressful, and they are chronic. They just can't go away! Most are beyond our control, and we are faced with the challenge to learn how to live with them in ways that minimize the distress we experience.

- In this session you will: (1) identify those chronic stressors in your life that box you in, (2) examine them thoroughly and (3) determine what you want to do with them (or in spite of them).

B. GUIDED FANTASY AND DRAWING (15 minutes)

2) The trainer reads the **Getting out of My Box** script which leads participants through an exploration of their personal boxes.

   ☞ *Tell people you are going to take them on a mental adventure. Encourage them to get comfortable, close their eyes, and begin relaxing. Some will want to lie on the floor or lean against the wall, others may remain in their chairs. You may want to turn down the lights just a bit (down, not off!).*

   *Be sure that people have the **My Personal Box** worksheet with them before they begin the fantasy trip. This will minimize disruption in the room after the fantasy when they are asked to draw their boxes.*

   You may wish to play some soft, reflective music in the background as you read the fantasy trip script. Read the script slowly, with ample pauses that allow participants time to image what you have suggested! Take 10 minutes to read this!

GETTING OUT OF MY BOX SCRIPT

Begin to become quiet within yourself . . .
   listen to your insides . . .
   relax . . . and concentrate on the steady . . .
   deep . . . rhythm of your breathing . . .

When you breathe in . . . fill yourself with air . . .
   fill you belly with air . . . expand . . .

When you breathe out . . . let yourself collapse . . .
   from the inside . . . like a balloon . . .
   with the air . . . going out . . .

Imagine you are taking a walk . . .
   on a beautiful path . . . on a green hillside . . .
   a setting like the Sound of Music . . .
   beautiful green hills . . .

As you walk . . . along the path . . .
   you notice some flowers . . . by the wayside . . .

You feel . . . the breeze on your face . . .
   you are at peace . . . and free . . .
   and enjoying yourself . . .

As you walk . . . you come to a fork in the path . . .
   one path goes right . . . one goes left . . .
   one is stony . . . and edged with grass . . .
   the other is wide . . . with a smooth surface . . .

You take one of those paths . . . and continue your walk . . .

As your walk continues . . .
   you notice you are approaching . . . a woods . . .

You come closer . . . and notice the trees . . .
   you keep walking . . . and enter the forest . . .

As you walk . . . the forest grows thicker . . .
   the light becomes dimmer . . .
   the greens rich and dark . . . the air cool . . .

As you continue . . . to walk in the forest . . .
  you notice a box . . . on the side of the path . . .

You stop . . . and you look . . .
  carefully noticing the details of this box . . .

And you look carefully at the box . . .
  noticing its size . . . and its shape . . . and its color . . .
  and you walk around it . . . slowly . . .
  noticing how it is made . . .

Then . . . just for fun . . .
  you decide . . . to try crawling . . . into the box . . .

You crawl in . . . and look at the inside . . . of the box . . .
  and notice the colors . . . the shapes . . .
  the smells . . . inside of the box . . .

You experiment by shutting the door to the box . . .
  shutting it slowly . . . so the light slowly fades . . .

You close it slowly . . . you close it completely . . .
  and see the crack of light . . . slowly fade and disappear . . .
  as the door shuts completely . . .

Now you are inside the box . . .
  and it is dark . . . and you are still . . .
  and you notice how you feel . . .

You notice the size of the box inside . . .
  you notice whether you want to sit quietly . . .
  or move . . . exploring the corners of the box . . .

You notice the quiet in the box . . .
  and you notice how you feel . . .

Soon . . . you realize that you are ready . . .
  to leave the box . . .

It is now time to escape . . .
  imagine how you escape . . . what do you try first? . . .
  where do you push? . . . how hard? . . . how long? . . .

Now you are out . . . you have escaped from the box . . .
  you notice your feelings . . .
  and you think back over the effort . . .
  of leaving . . . the box . . .
  and how you escaped . . .

Now you are outside the box . . .
once again in the light of the forest . . .
and you notice the sounds . . . and the feelings . . .

And you walk around the box once again . . .
checking it out . . . carefully . . .
so you can remember . . . all the details

How is it sitting? . . .
is it still the way it was when you found it? . . .
or has it moved? . . .

Is it still intact? . . .
or have the sides been broken out? . . .

You notice . . . and remember . . .
then you prepare yourself . . . to say good-bye . . .
to the box . . .

Because it is now time to move on . . .
but you keep the clear memory . . . of your experience . . .
with you . . . as you walk away . . . from the box . . .

And you walk . . . down the path . . .
only a short distance . . .
before you come out of the woods . . .
back into the bright sunlight . . . of the day . . .

And you come out of your journey . . .
back into the bright sunlight . . . of this room . . .

And you slowly . . . come out of your journey . . .
back into this room . . .

Carrying with you . . . back into this room . . .
the clear memory . . . of your box . . .
and your experience . . . with it . . .

As you come back into this room . . .
come back just far enough . . .
to take your worksheet and begin drawing a picture . . .
of your box . . .

Come back to this room . . .
pick up your worksheet . . . and start drawing your box . . .

Recall and draw all the details you can . . .
pay attention to the size . . . and color . . .
the construction . . . the shape . . .

©1983 Whole Person Press PO Box 3151 Duluth MN 55812   (218) 728-6807

*Note how the box was when you saw it first . . .
and how it was when you left it . . .*

*Recall how it felt for you . . .
on the outside . . . and on the inside . . .*

Embellish your drawing with all the details you can . . .

☞ *Allow 2–4 minutes for participants to draw their boxes.*

C. REFLECTION AND DIALOGUE (10–15 minutes)

3) After everyone has completed their drawings, the trainer helps participants focus on their boxes.

✔ What was the size of the box compared to you? Small and cramped? Big and roomy?

✔ How did you feel when you were inside the box? List two or three feeling words. Some of you may have felt panicky and wanted out fast. Others probably felt relaxed and quiet, comforted, protected.

✔ How did you escape? Did the door just open easily? Or did it lock? Did you get out easily or have to smash your way out? Or find the trick latch?

✔ How did you feel after you got out of the box? When you saw daylight again? When you knew you were still on your path? When you walked around it?

✔ How did you feel when you had to say "good-bye" to the box and leave it there as you moved on down the path? Did you miss it at all?

4) The trainer asks participants to focus on the meaning of their box fantasy, and introduces the dialogue.

➤ Look again at your box . . . and consider its meaning . . .

➤ Every person experiences factors in life that impinge on them, that hold them back, that put restrictions on their life, that squeeze them, control them and limit them.

➤ What are some of the factors in your life right now that you know are boxing you in? List a few! List whatever images come to your mind. (2 minutes)

➤ Look these over. Are there any common themes? Circle one that you'd like to focus on for the rest of this experience. Then let your box stand for this chronic stressor — give your box a name — label it.

➤ Take a moment to imagine that the picture of your box represents your chronic stressor.

➤ Now, I'd like you to hold a conversation with your box and record it in the space provided on the worksheet. Here's how you should begin:

> Write your dialogue with your box like a play . . . let your box speak to you first . . .

Box: "I am ___(your problem)___ and here's something I've got to say to you: _____."
You: " _____(write your response)_____ ."
Box: " _____(etc)_____ ."

➤ Everyone should start with *"I am your box . . . "* and then let the conversation flow from there. Don't try to guide the discussion or steer it in a particular direction. Rather, follow it! Listen to your chronic problem, hear what it has to say, then respond. You may end up arguing with your box or complimenting your box, or it may end up confronting you.

➤ Tell your box how you feel about it. Let your box tell you what it's doing for you or how it feels about you or how it feels about how you treat it! Be honest and direct — blunt if you need to be. Write as fast and as much as you can. Do not go back and read what you wrote! Just get started and see where you go.

☞ *Allow approximately 5 minutes for writing the dialogue. When there are about 30 seconds left, the trainer should ask people to write one more exchange using the format:*

Box: "Oh, yes — one more thing I want to tell you before I get cut off is: _____ ."
You: "Well — there is one last thing I have got to say to you _____ ."

6) In summary, the trainer asks participants to review their dialogues.

➤ Now, look over your dialogue. Read it. Notice the themes that have come up. What's happening? What are the feelings?

➤ Write down a couple of observations/insights/surprises that you notice about your dialogue and your relationship with your box.

D. INTERPERSONAL DIALOGUE (20–30 minutes)

7) The trainer divides participants into groups of 4 persons each, or utilizes previously established sharing units, and instructs participants to share with each other their experience in this exercise.

➤ Spend the first 10 minutes describing the initial experience with your box on the fantasy trip and showing each other your pictures.

➤ Then you should take 4–5 minutes each to:
> describe the chronic stressor that your box came to symbolize for you
> read your dialogue (this is essential!) and
> share your insights and observations regarding its meaning.

8) After about 25 minutes, the trainer reconvenes the total group and invites comments and observations.

E. RESOLUTIONS FOR CHANGE (10 minutes)

9) The trainer leads participants through the second half of the worksheet entitled *Why My Box May Be a Good Place,* amplifying each point and giving participants time to write their answers before moving on to the next item.

● **Every box offers some positive reward in addition to its pain.** Examples:
* Financial rewards may make a high stress job worth doing.
* Eating too much offers a sedative for reducing tension.
* If I'm ill, others may reach out and "take care of me."

➤ *What are the positive rewards that you receive by staying locked in your box?* Record your answers on the *Why My Box May Be a Good Place* worksheet.

● **Every box also offers indirect rewards, since it offers you a chance to avoid other fearful situations.** Examples:
* Staying in a difficult relationship offers the comfort that you don't have to be on your own right now.
* Physical limitations may be "an excuse with honor" to avoid competing in the rat race.

* Perfectionist expectations ("If I can't do it perfectly, I won't do it at all.") allow you to avoid even trying.

➤ *What do you avoid by staying in your box?* Again, record your answers on the worksheet.

● **Every box, no matter how awful and painful, offers the comfort of the known** instead of the fear of the unknown. Examples:

　　* Staying in a deadend job may be better than facing potential failure in a more challenging position.

　　* Remaining chronically disappointed in a relationship may be better than finding a way to get what you want and then discovering that it wasn't what you wanted after all.

➤ *When you consider leaving your box behind you, what do you fear?* Jot down your fears on your worksheet.

10) Following the completion of these questions, participants, are instructed to summarize their mixed feelings about their boxes by completing the *Should I Make a Change* section of the worksheet, listing reasons for and reasons against making a change.

11) Finally, the trainer directs participants to write a summary of the changes they would like to make — in themselves and/or in their box.

🖝 *Be sure to remind people that they probably do not want to totally destroy their box. More likely, they want to reshape it in some way so they minimize the chronic pain but maintain some of the rewards. Encourage participants to be as specific as possible.*

F. SMALL AND LARGE GROUP SHARING (15–20 minutes)

12) The trainer asks participants to return to their sharing groups and spend 15–20 minutes summarizing their insights and resolutions.

13) The trainer reconvenes the total group and asks for a sharing of observations/insights/specific examples. In the ensuing discussion the trainer may wish to highlight some or all of the following points.

- Our "boxes" always bring with them a mixture of pain we'd like to avoid, along with rewards and comforts we'd liked to keep.

- **We seldom totally get rid of chronic problems**. They're called chronic because they are. If you've tried to get rid of the problem month after month, year after year, and it hasn't budged, perhaps it's here with you to stay.

- It's not so terrible to experience chronic problems. The American dream of a perfect, pain-free life is an illusion. **Everyone must live with some limitations**, chronic disappointments, and nagging stressors that we call "boxes".

  Many great figures in history have been great because they learned how to live with and rise above their personal "boxes" — not because they figured out how to live problem-free lives.

- Instead of trying to get rid of all your chronic stressors, you might better ask, "Given all these difficult and disappointing limitations in my life, **what must I do to take better care of myself?**" There's always something you can do to nurture yourself if you'll spend less time trying to get rid of problems and more time simply taking better care of yourself.

- **Every problem is a teacher**. Your "thorn in the flesh" will deepen your understanding of life, enhance your compassion, expand your faith, if you will only ask yourself, "What is it I can learn about life from this?" — and then listen to the answer.

- **You and your problems are not the same**. You are more than your problems. Your identity as a person is separate from your pain.

- No matter what limitations entrap you — no matter what disappointments box you in — you are still lovable. Nothing is ever so bad that it makes you worthless. God will love you if you will only allow it. Others will love you if you will only accept it. You can still love yourself if you are willing! Don't sell yourself a bill of goods, **you don't have to be perfect to be loved!**

VARIATIONS

- This exercise could be supplemented with a more extended planning process that helps participants identify desired change and formulate a program for enhancing it.

- If time is short, one of the two small group discussions could be eliminated. However, participants may feel somewhat overwhelmed by the amount of self-reflection they are asked to do if they don't have enough air time to share their experience and insights.

TRAINER'S NOTES

*This exercise was adapted from a program entitled **Dealing with Chronically Stressful Situations** designed and presented jointly by Alice Floreen and Don Tubesing at Miller Dwan Hospital, Duluth MN.*

MY PERSONAL BOX

MY DIALOGUE WITH MY BOX

WHY MY BOX MAY BE A GOOD PLACE

1) Positive rewards for staying there:

2) Things I avoid by being there:

3) What I fear about changing my box:

SHOULD I MAKE A CHANGE?
Yes, *because:*   *No*, *because:*

CHANGES I'D LIKE TO MAKE:
in me: *in my box:*

©1983 Whole Person Press PO Box 3151 Duluth MN 55812   (218) 728-6807

22 ONE STEP AT A TIME

This nine part guide leads participants step-by-step through a creative planning process for coping with a stress-related problem.

GOALS

To subject at least one stress-related problem to a comprehensive planning approach.

To encourage creativity in action planning.

To elicit personal commitment to change.

GROUP SIZE
Unlimited; works equally well with individuals.

TIME FRAME
20–30 minutes

MATERIALS NEEDED
A **Nine Step Planning Guide** worksheet for each participant.

PROCESS
1) The trainer invites participants to switch gears from "taking in" information to "sorting out" what they've learned and applying those insights to a specific stress-related problem. He distributes copies of the **Nine Step Planning Guide** to the group.

2) The trainer leads participants through the planning guide.

> ☞ *This planning process works best when the trainer controls the pacing. He should talk participants through the guide, reading the first question, giving examples where appropriate, pausing long enough for most people to answer the question before moving on to the next question and repeating the process.*

> *Some participants may have difficulty with the ambiguity of some questions. Clarify as necessary, but also remind people that this process is designed to tap into their own internal wisdom and meaning system.*

3) When everyone has finished, the trainer asks for volunteers to share their plans briefly with the group.

VARIATION
- After completing the seventh planning step, participants could divide into small groups (3–4 persons) to share their plans. The groups could then assist each member in brainstorming creative modifications and possible rewards. Add 20 minutes.

TRAINER'S NOTES

*Adapted from Donald A Tubesing, **Kicking Your Stress Habits**, (Duluth MN: Whole Person Associates, 1981).*

NINE STEP PLANNING GUIDE

This guide will lead you step-by-step through a creative planning process for coping with stress. It draws on your internal wisdom, so spend more time on the questions that strike you as particularly meaningful.

1 SUMMARIZE YOUR SYMPTOMS

What is wrong? Where are you experiencing pain? What are you worried about? What signals are indicating stress in your life?

2 DEFINE THE PROBLEM FROM SEVERAL PERSPECTIVES

What is the source of your stress? Write three or four different descriptions of the problem. Which one most clearly captures the cause of your stress?

1)

2)

3)

4)

3 LEARN FROM PREVIOUS PROBLEM-SOLVING ATTEMPTS

What coping strategies have you already tried? Why didn't they work? What new strategies are suggested by these previous failures?

4 CHECK YOUR ATTITUDE

How do you feel about this problem and your capability to deal with it?

____ hopeless ____ doubtful ____ maybe ____ possible ____ hopeful

What about your desire to tackle the problem and do something about it?

____ not motivated   ____ willing to try
____ partially committed   ____ highly motivated

5 IDENTIFY YOUR RESOURCES

What special strengths and skills can you bring to bear on the problem? Who will support you in the process?

6 SPECIFY YOUR GOALS

What do you want to happen? To feel? To change? To accomplish? To increase or decrease? To learn? Be very specific.

I want _____

I want _____

I want _____

I want _____

I want _____

I want _____

Go back now and review your goals. What would you have to give up in order to reach them? Are you willing to make this sacrifice? Are there some aspects of your problem you'd rather not change right now? What movement do you want to make?

7 FORMULATE A CLEAR PLAN OF ACTION

Based on the changes you want to make and the goals you've set, what specifically can you do?

I could _____

I could _____

I could _____

I could _____

I could _____

I could _____

I could _____

I could _____

I could _____

Go back and rate each of these potential action plans according to these criteria:
>   1) Is it specific?
>   2) Does it avoid radical change?
>   3) Does it have long-term value?
>   4) Will it provide some secondary benefits?
>   5) Does it involve you as a whole person?

Now, what exactly will you plan to do? Include details on frequency, starting point, ending point, etc.

I will _____

I will _____

I will _____

I will _____

I will _____

I will _____

I will _____

I will _____

8 ADD A CREATIVE TOUCH

Creativity makes any plan more enjoyable — and usually more successful. How could you spice up your commitment?
Exaggerate it? Do it backwards? Minimize it?
Combine it with something? Complicate it?
Do it with a friend? Do it at a different time?

9 REWARD YOURSELF

What special treats will you give yourself when you accomplish some or all of your plan?

23 POSTSCRIPT

In this action planning exercise participants write themselves letters which are then collected by the trainer and mailed sometime later as a reminder of the learning that took place.

GOALS

To structure integrative thinking about stress management goals and issues.

To provide a long-term link between the learning experience and the participants' daily living.

GROUP SIZE

Any size group is appropriate, as the work is done individually.

TIME FRAME

15 minutes

MATERIALS NEEDED

Blank paper and an envelope for each participant.

PROCESS

1) The trainer distributes an envelope to each participant and asks them to write their own name and mailing address on their envelope.

2) The trainer describes the letter-writing and follow-up process. (Participants will write a letter about self-care to themselves, put it in an envelope and return it to the trainer. At some future date, the trainer will mail the envelopes to the participants.)

   ☞ *Typically groups appreciate this little joke: "Sometime in the future you will go get your mail and exclaim to yourself, 'My gosh, there's someone out there who has handwriting just like mine!!'"*

3) The trainer guides participants through the letter-writing, adapting the content to fit the emphasis of the learning experience. A typical letter would include the following elements:

➤ Date and salutation.

➤ A short paragraph or a list of statements, symbols, etc, regarding the ways in which participants *already* manage their stress in healthy, adaptive ways.

> ☞ *Since this letter is for the participant's personal use, the style in which it is done is far less important than the fact that each person is doing it!*

➤ A paragraph outlining the stress management skills that they will be adding to their repertoire and practicing over the next several months.

➤ A paragraph listing important members of the participant's support system, as well as other persons worth adding to that support system in the months ahead.

➤ A final paragraph noting any thoughts or reflections about the learning experience that will be important to recall in the future.

4) The trainer has each participant seal the letter into the envelope, then collects them.

5) One to six months later the trainer mails the envelopes to participants.

VARIATIONS

■ Content of the letter can vary significantly to reflect the nature of the learning experience and the needs of the participants. Letters from an organizational training session, for example, could focus on balancing personal self-care with contributions to organizational improvement.

■ Form letters with a listing of the issues to be addressed or with sentence stems could be used instead of the trainer-directed process.

Contributed by Tim Hatfield, who first experienced this adaptation of an old stand-by during a life and career planning workshop led by Janet Hagberg of Minneapolis MN.

24 COPING SKILL AFFIRMATION

This exercise is designed to affirm participants' positive stress management coping skills, and is most effective at the conclusion of an ongoing learning experience.

GOALS

To stimulate specific thinking about participants' own coping skills.

To provide an opportunity to affirm the positive coping skills of oneself and others.

To structure a situation in which participants receive significant affirmations from others with whom they have been interacting.

GROUP SIZE

Designed for use in groups of 4 to 8 persons who have been an intact sharing/work group for a significant portion of the overall learning experience (ie, it will be non-productive or counter-productive for groups of persons who do not know each other).

TIME FRAME

60 minutes

MATERIALS NEEDED

Ample 3x5 note cards or small pieces of scratch paper.

PROCESS

1) The trainer begins the exercise by reiterating to the participants that they have, as individuals, a variety of adaptive coping skills with which to confront the inevitable stresses of everyday living.

2) The trainer distributes note cards or scratch paper to each small group.

   ☞ *Each group should receive a certain number of note cards, based on the size of the group.*

☞ *4 persons: 12 cards each, total 48 per group*
5 persons: 15 cards each, total 75 per group
6 persons: 15 card each, total 90 per group
7 persons: 21 cards each, total 147 per group
8 persons: 24 cards each, total 192 per group

➤ Focus on one person at a time. Take three cards and write the person's name on the card.

➤ Identify the **three most significant stress management skills** you see in that group member and write one skill on each of her cards. Repeat this process for each member of your group. You will end up with three skill cards for everyone.

3) Working individually, each group member writes on scrap paper all the ways in which he *successfully* and *positively* manages the stress in his life. The more ideas the better. (5 minutes)

4) The trainer asks each participant to put his name on three note cards. He then selects the three most important stress management skills from his original list and writes them, one skill per note card on the three labeled cards. These cards are temporarily set aside.

5) Next the trainer instructs the participants to make a similar set of three skill affirmation cards for each member of his small group.(10–15 minutes)

6) The trainer describes the process for sharing affirmations in the small group. One person volunteers to be "it" — the receiver — first. One-by-one the other group members read the skills they have chosen to affirm for the receiver, handing the note cards to the receiver as they read them.

The trainer outlines special "rules" for the exchange.

➤ **For the person receiving messages** — you are to listen only. No second-guessing, no "yes-buts", no explanations, no wiping out the gifts you are receiving. It is OK, however, to thank the giver of the three messages after he is finished.

➤ **For the person giving messages** — you are to speak directly to the person whose skills you are affirming. Read each card giving examples of times when you have observed her using that skill. Look at the person; give your gifts directly.

➤ **For the other group members** — pay attention to the gift giving. Please don't talk. Observe carefully and listen respectfully.

☞ *Announce that this process will take 30 minutes or more —*
and will be well worth the time.

7) After the affirmation process is completed, the trainer may
gather the groups back together and close the learning
experience by asking for affirmation from participants of what
they have learned or qualities they have appreciated in the
trainer.

☞ *Don't pass by this opportunity to practice receiving gifts*
from those to whom you have given so much. Although this
may seem hokey — most groups appreciate the opportunity
to affirm the trainer. Be sure you observe the rules —
accept the comments and limit yourself to a "thank you" in
return. This process will leave everyone with a warm glow
at the end of the learning experience.

VARIATION

■ Although it certainly would be possible to do this exercise
verbally (with none of the writing and handing over of
messages), the additional structure helps keep people on track
while providing participants with some tangible, concrete
affirming messages to save as a reminder of the learning
experience.

TRAINER'S NOTES

Submitted by Tim Hatfield

GROUP ENERGIZERS

25 BOO-DOWN

This quick exercise exposes the role of irrational beliefs in creating stress and actively engages the entire group in laughing at the stupidity of unreasonable standards and expectations.

GOALS
To help participants deal with irrational beliefs at a conscious, rather than unconscious level.

To demonstrate how beliefs can cause stress.

GROUP SIZE
Unlimited; works especially well in large groups.

TIME FRAME
5 minutes

MATERIALS NEEDED
One set of **Irrational Belief Cards**

PROCESS

☞ *The trainer will need to prepare a deck of **Irrational Belief Cards** using the suggestions on page 115.*

1) The trainer describes the functioning of our belief system and its role in creating stress. She notes that irrational beliefs are sneaky. They do their work under cover, where they're hardly recognized.

   The trainer explains that this exercise will help participants bring the irrational beliefs out in the open where their foolishness becomes immediately obvious.

2) The trainer asks (assigns) 6–8 volunteers to come to the microphone. Each is handed one of the **Irrational Belief Cards** and told to prepare for reading the card to the group with intensity and feeling.

3) The participants in the "audience" are instructed to be at their cynical best. As each card is read, they are to hiss, boo, laugh,

jeer, make caustic comments, etc. In any and every way, they are to ridicule the belief.

4) One at a time, volunteers read "their" irrational belief and the group responds with a *boo-down*.

☞ *Keep this process moving. Let the reading and response take the form of a litany, and let the pace build in intensity to a crashing crescendo at the end.*

✔ The trainer asks, "Does anyone recognize any of these messages?"

VARIATIONS

■ This energizer is a good warm-up or wrap-up for an exercise that engages participants in identifying and disputing their own irrational belief systems.

■ Instead of utilizing the **Irrational Belief Cards** provided, the trainer may prefer to write out a set of irrational beliefs specific to the issues of the participant group, and/or the topic/problem area being discussed. For example, some personalized beliefs for nurses might read:

I must be competent — absolutely without fault
— in everything I do.
If I'm going to do it — then I'll do it better
than anyone else . . . whatever it is . . .

I must be a **perfect** – med/surg nurse . . .
perfect – in emergencies . . .
a **perfect** – listener when people want to talk . . .
a **perfect** – administrator and planner.

And when I'm off duty – I must also be . . .
perfect – as a friend, parent, spouse and lover.

Whenever I'm not Superwoman/Superman I'm disappointed in myself.
I don't like feeling disappointed.
I have just got to be the best!

■ The belief statements from *Lifetrap 1: Workaholism (Stress 1, p 47)* would make an excellent boo-down litany.

The process of this exercise was suggested by Rev William E Peterson MSW, Wholistic Health Centers Inc, Hinsdale IL.

IRRATIONAL BELIEF CARDS

You people are too strong and confident. I am so weak,
I do dumb things — like standing up here right now!
I can't do much on my own — that's why I'm reading this speech!
You do things so much better than I do.
You are so good at everything.
I need you to take care of me . . . Please!

If I didn't have such a crummy past,
I would amount to a whole lot more these days.
My parents gave me a bad start
and life just hasn't given me much of a chance!

If I don't do what others want, they won't like me.
If I refuse, they will be angry.
I owe it to others to do what they want.
So I always say "yes" to keep them happy!

Some of the mean, ugly people in my life cause
me a lot of grief.
I try to be patient and understanding but I must say that
*often when I'm unhappy, it's **really other peoples' fault!***
If I could only get rid of those people
I'd be a whole lot better off.

If I don't reach all of the goals I set for myself,
I'm not worth much as a person!

I'd be happier if I didn't have to worry so much.
I am anxious about all kinds of problems.
These problems keep me from being happy.
Unless I get rid of them, I'll always be a basket case!
And I'll never be happy.

It is terribly important to me that everyone likes me
— all of the time!
And that everyone is always satisfied with everything I do.
Everyone needs to love me and approve of me all of the time.
I hope you like what I've just said
— because I want all of you to be pleased with me too!

Every problem has a right answer and solution
— all other solutions are wrong.
No matter what the issue, I can figure out how to fix
everything. Give me time and I'll find the right answer.

©1983 Whole Person Press PO Box 3151 Duluth MN 55812   (218) 728-6807

26 BREATH-LESS

This highly effective tool confronts participants with the need to breathe properly.

GOALS

To demonstrate that under pressure most people forget to breathe deeply.

To provoke discussion about the importance of relaxation as a coping skill.

TIME FRAME

2 minutes

PROCESS

1) The trainer makes a brief presentation highlighting the importance of consistent deep breathing and noting its relaxation effect on the entire body through parasympathetic rebound. The trainer explains that sometimes (especially in stressful situations) we actually forget to breathe, which robs our body of its oxygen supply, de-energizes us, and diminishes our effectiveness in dealing with stress.

2) The trainer asks participants to stand and instructs them to look, on the count of "1", at a designated spot on the right side of the room. On the count of "2" they will shift their *eyes only* to a designated spot on the left side of the room. Participants are not to move their heads.

3) The trainer says, "That's simple enough. Now, go! One . . . Two . . . One . . . Two . . . One . . . Two . . . Stop!"

4) The trainer observes that no one has been breathing during the exercise. The intense concentration and anxiety over following directions has taken precedence over normal breathing processes.

5) The trainer facilitates further discussion of the importance of breathing.

Submitted by Sandy Queen

27 CATASTROPHE GAME

Participants take turns exaggerating their stressful life situations into major catastrophes, discovering in the process the absurdity of their "awfulizing" habits.

GOALS
To highlight the assets and liabilities of complaining as a stress management technique.

TIME FRAME
10–15 minutes

PROCESS
1) The trainer asks participants to make a quick list of the stressors that are active in their lives right now. What problems are troubling them? What difficult situations are surrounding them? (1 minute)

2) Participants pair up with a neighbor and start catastrophizing. The first person chooses a stressful incident and describes what happened, dramatizing the scene and exaggerating the unpleasant feelings.

   After a minute or two, the second person gets a chance to top that story! He chooses a stressor of his own and starts catastrophizing. As soon as he's done, the first person picks another stressor and starts complaining again.

   Pairs continue awfulizing, each one trying to top the other's catastrophe, until the trainer calls time. (5–10 minutes)

   ☞ *The energy in the room usually increases dramatically during this routine. It's often tough to get people to stop catastrophizing.*

3) The trainer reconvenes the group and comments on complaining as a stress management strategy.

   ● **Complaining can be an energizer.** Like alcohol, it is effective in small doses for tension-reducing — but in the long run it's a dead-end unless it leads to some positive change.

- **Catastrophizing can be a coping skill** if it helps us see how we've exaggerated little irritants into big annoyances. If we can laugh at ourselves, we've already taken a positive step toward managing our stress.

- The final "play" in the catastrophe game is to ask and answer the question: "In the midst of all this chaos (pain/anxiety/trouble), **how can I take care of myself?**"

VARIATIONS

- The catastrophe game theme could be easily altered to fit specific learning objectives. Participants might catastrophize about "awful working conditions" or "all the things I'm worried about" or "all the expectations others have of me," etc. Any of the irrational beliefs in *Boo-Down (Stress 1, p 113)* would make good subjects for catastrophizing.

- In addition to describing their catastrophe in *Step 2*, participants could also imagine all kinds of other things that might go wrong to make the situation even worse, then elaborate on the possible consequences.

TRAINER'S NOTES

28 FRUIT BASKET UPSET

Participants find a new spot in the room and a new outlook on their stress.

GOALS

To heighten awareness of the power of perception in stress management.

TIME FRAME

2–5 minutes

PROCESS

1) The trainer describes briefly the role of perception in creating stress and relieving it as well. He asks participants to join an *in vivo* demonstration of the impact of a new outlook.

2) Participants pick up their belongings and move to a new space in the room which offers a different perspective.

3) After the next teaching segment the trainer invites participants to comment on what they experienced by changing perspective.

29 GET OFF MY BACK!

Participants symbolically shrug off their troubles in this loud and lively self-assertiveness exercise.

GOALS

To raise participants' awareness of the stresses and strains that weigh them down.

To practice a whole person un-burdening process.

TIME FRAME

2 minutes

PROCESS

1) The trainer directs participants to slump in their chairs, as if they were carrying a heavy weight on their shoulders/back.

2) Once everyone has assumed the "bowed down" posture, the trainer asks people to think of all the burdens they're carrying around these days — all the worries and concerns, the stresses and strains, the trials and tribulations.

    ☞ *The trainer will probably want to give several examples and suggest that most people are carrying around a lot of extra burdens that aren't even their own.*

    Participants mentally visualize and name each of the burdens and imagine them as part of the weight on their back.

3) At a signal from the trainer, participants leap out of their chairs, with arms outstretched, shouting in unison, *Get Off My Back!*

4) The trainer invites participants to try it again, and again — until the group energy level rises and the individual tension levels diminish.

5) The trainer concludes with the observation that many people — especially folks in "helping" roles — confuse *caring* for others with *carrying* their burdens.

We learned this exercise at a burnout workshop conducted by Judy and Tom Wright, Minneapolis MN.

©1983 Whole Person Press PO Box 3151 Duluth MN 55812   (218) 728-6807

30 HOT POTATO PROBLEM

This exercise engages participants in a humorous process of defining and dealing with a shared group stressor. It is especially effective with intact groups who live or work together.

GOALS

To help participants openly identify a common stressor.

To graphically demonstrate the natural tendency to "pass the buck" and blame others.

To illustrate the dysfunctional nature of scapegoating as a problem-solving technique.

GROUP SIZE

Unlimited

TIME FRAME

20–30 minutes

MATERIALS NEEDED

Tape recorder/record player/piano player and music; groups choose a physical symbol for their problem from whatever objects are available in the room.

PROCESS

☞ *If the group is small and homogenous, the trainer may want to keep everyone together as a work team for this exercise. With larger or more diverse groups, she should divide participants into work teams of 6–10 persons each.*

1) The trainer divides participants into work teams.

2) The trainer instructs the participants of each team to identify a distress-causing issue common to everyone in their group. (3–5 minutes)

3) Each team selects some physical item from the room that will symbolize their common stressor. Participants vocally christen their "hot potato" with the name of their problem.

☞ *This item will be the group's hot potato — it must be small enough to be handled easily and passed back and forth.*

The trainer describes the rules of the Hot Potato Game.

➤ One participant holds the hot potato.

➤ When the music begins that participant is to say, **"This (name of problem) is not mine. It is yours, (name of recipient)."** The potato is passed to the recipient. (It can be rolled, thrown, or handed over.)

➤ The new recipient must redefine the problem and give it a slightly new label before passing it on. If no new label is offered, the participant gets the problem back, and must hold it until he finds some way to redefine it.

The words go like this: **No, the problem isn't (old name), really it is (new name). And, (name of next recipient), it is now yours".**

Again, the hot potato is passed.

➤ As long as the music plays, the problem continues to be redefined and passed. However, it cannot be passed to any participant the second time until all have received it once.

➤ When the music stops, the group verbally scapegoats the one holding the problem, and that person is out of the game — becoming an observer for the succeeding rounds.

➤ Rounds of music, problem passing, and scapegoating are continued until only the "winner" remains. That survivor now must accept full responsibility for dealing with the group's problem alone, being the only remaining member still active. The "winner" gets to keep the problem and do with it as he likes, but must publicly accept full ownership of the problem.

5) The group (or small groups) discuss their reactions to the process. They analyze the "effectiveness" of "passing the buck" and scapegoating, and explore the meaning of the game's result — namely that the "winner" in the Hot Potato Game ultimately ends up alone, to deal with the problem in isolation.

6) The trainer invites a sharing of observations and insights. The trainer discusses alternate problem-solving methods based on joint ownership of the problem that will lead to more positive long-term results.

VARIATIONS

■ With an intact work group this exercise could be followed with a problem-solving process applied to the common stressor.

■ This exercise is adaptable for use in stress-producing, conflict-laden situations in marriage or family relationships, especially when family members are prone to blame each other for their difficulties.

■ In an alternate approach, the participant "left holding the problem" must stand and publicly acknowledge it as his own, and then briefly carry it around the room as a burden.

TRAINER'S NOTES

31 PULLING STRINGS

In this relaxing exercise participants pretend they are marionettes and allow their bodies to loosen up as they move around the room.

GOALS

To experience the sensation of voluntary letting go of muscular tension.

GROUP SIZE

Unlimited as long as there is plenty of space to move around.

TIME FRAME

5–10 minutes

PROCESS

1) The trainer introduces the exercise, explaining that it is designed to help them limber up and let go of the tension they have accumulated during the day.

2) Participants stand and spread themselves throughout the room. Each person needs at least a three foot square of turf.

3) The trainer directs people to imagine they are marionettes (like Pinocchio), with strings attached to their knees, wrists and head. They are to let the muscles of their body go limp and floppy, as if suspended by strings at these three points. The trainer demonstrates the position.

4) The trainer directs participants to perform a variety of actions in the way they imagine a marionette would do them, reminding everyone to stay loose and relaxed throughout.

    ☞ *The trainer can have fun dreaming up appropriate actions. Start with something simple like walking a few steps or clapping hands. Then progress to more complicated maneuvers such as jumping jacks, riding on a subway, climbing on a bike, picking up something from the floor, or hugging another participant. Work activities are fun to pantomime and provide models for on-the-job relaxation.*

32 SINGALONG 2

Participants join in two "ditties with a message" set to familiar melodies.

GOALS

To encourage participants to laugh at their stress-producing thinking habits.

To reinforce less stress-provoking attitudes/beliefs.

GROUP SIZE

Unlimited

TIME FRAME

2–5 minutes

MATERIALS NEEDED

Blackboard, newsprint easel or copies of the *Stress Theme Songs*.

PROCESS

1) The trainer chooses one or more of the stress theme songs and teaches it to the group.

   ☞ *The trainer may want to distribute copies of the songs to all participants or write the lyrics on the blackboard or newsprint.*

   If the group is not familiar with the "Funiculi, Funicula" tune, ask those who know the song to teach the others by singing it through once or twice.

2) For the *Stress Yourself* song, the group should sing it through in unison once or twice, then divide into four sections for singing in rounds. Each section sings the song through three times.

   ☞ *The last line of this song can easily be replaced with a different message such as "Now's the time to play," or "Headache on the way." Make up your own or invite the group to brainstorm alternatives.*

©1983 Whole Person Press PO Box 3151 Duluth MN 55812   (218) 728-6807

STRESS THEME SONGS

STRESS YOURSELF
(sung to the tune of "Row, Row, Row Your Boat")

Stress, stress, stress yourself
All throughout the day —
Verily, verily, verily, verily
Distress on the way!

TYPE A THEME SONG
(sung to the tune of "Funiculi, Funicula")

Some think the world was made for fun and frolic.
But, oh not I! but, oh not I!
I think it best to be a workaholic.
To do or die, to do or die.

I, I like to spend my life succeeding
In many roles
With few controls.
Or else I occupy my time exceeding
My short range goals,
My long range goals.

"Work Hard! Work Hard!" prods my inner voice.
"Hard Work! Hard work!" there is no other choice!

But if I drive myself so fast,
I know my heart will never last.
If I want to live,
I must slow down! I must relax!

Original lyrics by Nancy Loving Tubesing

©1983 Whole Person Press PO Box 3151 Duluth MN 55812   (218) 728-6807

33 STRESS SPENDING

Using the cash in their pockets as a symbol of time and energy investment in their stressors, participants illustrate their current stress spending patterns.

GOALS

To help participants identify the quantity of time and energy they are spending on their stressors.

To demonstrate that investment in stressors is a decision.

GROUP SIZE

Flexible, could also be used with individuals.

TIME FRAME

10–30 minutes

MATERIALS NEEDED

Table or floor space to spread out coins and several small pieces of paper for each participant.

PROCESS

1) The trainer asks participants to list several of their current stressors (at least 5–8), or refer back to a list created earlier in the seminar.

2) The trainer distributes several small pieces of paper to each person. Participants make a "name tag" for each stressor and spread these markers face up on the table in front of them.

3) Participants remove whatever cash they have with them from their wallets, pockets or purses and use it to represent their time and energy expenditure.

4) Each person divides his money among the stressor name tags in proportion to the amount of time and energy he is currently investing in each stressor.

©1983 Whole Person Press PO Box 3151 Duluth MN 55812   (218) 728-6807

5) Participants individually make notes to themselves on the surprises, insights and resolutions that occur to them as they observe their stress spending pattern.

6) The trainer invites the sharing of salient observations. In the ensuing discussion the trainer may wish to compare the spending patterns in the exercise with real life situations.

● **Spending priorities are different** for each person. During this exercise some people probably found that they are spending way too much of themselves on some issues and way too little on others.

The crucial question is, "Are my energy-spending priorities consistent with what I believe is really important?"

● **It's not "fair."** Participants started with differing amounts of cash — some a lot, others just a little. Some had more yesterday, but little left today. Some may be getting paid tomorrow!

That's the way it is with life! Some of us have more energy and resiliency than others. For each of us the extent of energy reserves we possess varies from day to day, from year to year, from one stage of life to the next. It's not fair! But it's true.

● **Investing in stress is a choice.** Some people used up all of their cash on their stress. Others held some back in reserve to spend on high-energy vitalizers or creative adventures yet to be discovered.

In the real world some people are willing to spend all of their time and energy on their stressful problems, too! Others are only willing to give part of themselves to their problems, preferring instead to save some of themselves for other life-issues.

Which style is likely to be more healthful in the long run?

VARIATIONS

■ Participants could place the money on their stressors twice — first, to represent their current spending pattern; second, to represent the way they think it *should* be.

■ The depth of this exercise could be enhanced by including small group sharing before or after *Step 6*. Participants show others their money placement (stress spending) pattern, describe their reactions and ask others in the group to comment on what they see.

34 STRETCH

In this fun-filled relaxation break participants stretch and limber the major muscle groups.

GOALS

To demonstrate a tension-relieving stretch routine.

To discharge accumulated tension.

GROUP SIZE

Unlimited as long as everyone has some space for movement.

TIME FRAME

5 minutes

PROCESS

1) The trainer invites participants to join in a refreshing stretch break. She directs people to stretch both arms up toward the ceiling with hands and fingers out-stretched . . . stretch . . . and then droop, relax, let go!

    ☞ *The trainer may want to reduce inhibitions by saying, "Don't worry — nobody's looking at your belly except me!"*

    Participants repeat the stretch.

2) The trainer comments that tension reduction is a serious issue in stress management — but with a little imagination relaxation can also be fun!

    The trainer demonstrates as she instructs participants to imagine they have a pencil on the tip of their chin and write the word *stretch* in the air.

    ☞ *Encourage people to use wide, sweeping movements that really stretch the neck and shoulder muscles.*

3) The trainer directs people to use the same process, this time writing their first name across the sky with the *right elbow*.

4) Next participants use the *left elbow* to write their last name — backwards!

5) The trainer asks participants to lower their focus a little and use the *left hip* to write their lover's name in big letters.

☞ *The trainer can comment, "Don't worry — no one will be able to read what you write!" People may need some extra encouragement here to loosen up and stretch their pelvic and back areas. Be sure to exaggerate your own movements when demonstrating.*

6) Finally, the trainer announces that for those people who think this exercise is silly and believe the group should be more serious, participants next use the *right hip* to write the Apostle's Creed (or Pledge of Allegiance or Hippocratic Oath or Company Policy and Procedure Manual, etc).

TRAINER'S NOTES

35 TEN GREAT TRIPS ON FOOT

Participants combine exercise with fantasy to take a delightful 5-minute mind-body vacation.

GOALS

To reinforce the importance of exercise as a stress management technique.

To increase motivation to exercise.

TIME FRAME

5 minutes

PROCESS

1) The trainer reviews the triple benefits of exercise as a strategy for dealing with stress.

- **Regular exercise strengthens us and increases our stamina** so that we are physically more capable to deal with the effects of stress.

- **Exercise is a natural tension reducer.** The profound relaxation that follows vigorous exercise is a great antidote to stress.

- **Many people find that exercise promotes mental stimulation** and tranquility as well as physical invigoration and relaxation.

2) The trainer invites participants to join in some mind-body exercise. He asks people to stand up and spread around in the room until everyone has space for free movement.

3) The trainer asks everyone to start slowly jogging or walking in place, announcing "We are going to run to some fun places — so close your eyes if you can and run along with me."

☞ *The trainer chooses one of the ten great trip visualizations and guides the group on the journey, adding lots of vivid imagery that promotes sensory awareness along the way. If there's time, take three or four different trips. Allow a minute or two for "cooling down" — after the trip.*

VARIATIONS

■ If space permits, the group could walk/jog around the room rather than staying in one place.

■ The trainer could make up his own visualizations, including some trips in and around the immediate locale. Try a jog through a nearby shopping mall or sewage plant. How about a brisk walk through downtown or down the aisle of the church or the corner? How about walking on water or Cloud 9?!

TRAINER'S NOTES

TEN GREAT TRIPS ON FOOT

1) You are running across the Golden Gate bridge with the bay breeze at your back . . .

2) You are running up the stairs at the Washington Monument . . .

3) You are the last person carrying the Olympic torch, striding down the runway into the stadium . . .

4) You have just reached the top of Heartbreak Hill in the Boston Marathon and feel a surge of energy as you start down the home stretch . . .

5) You are sprinting down the corridor at O'Hare airport trying to make the last plane home . . .

6) You are walking down the Bright Angel trail at the Grand Canyon . . .

7) You are just starting the traditional fifteen mile hike from camp to the nearest candy store . . .

8) You are jogging in the warm sand along the shore at sunset . . .

9) You are hiking in an alpine meadow; the sky is vivid blue and the gentle tinkle of cowbells surrounds you . . .

10) You are marching in the 4th of July parade. The band starts into its quick-step routine . . .

©1983 Whole Person Press PO Box 3151 Duluth MN 55812   (218) 728-6807

36 TENSION HURTS

In this thought-provoking exercise, participants learn first-hand about the relationship between tension and pain.

GOALS

To demonstrate the physical effects of chronic tension.

To motivate participants to learn and practice relaxation techniques.

TIME FRAME

5 minutes

PROCESS

1) The trainer points out that people under stress often experience chronic tension. She invites participants to demonstrate the fact that tension hurts.

2) Participants are directed to tightly clench their jaw or one fist. (2–3 minutes)

   ☞ *The trainer will need to keep reminding people to keep tensing the muscle, feeling the pain growing yet continuing to hold the tension until the time is up. If the trainer is doing the exercise with the group, her own pain level will probably be a good indication of when to stop. Don't stop too soon! The point is to experience the pain caused by tension.*

3) When most people are clearly feeling acute pain, the trainer instructs participants to let go — relax — and allow the pain to go away.

4) The trainer points out the moral of the story:

   - **Tension hurts**. Many of us experience pain in joints, muscles or organs that originates with chronic tension. Systematic relaxation can alleviate some of that tension and pain.

   - **The same principle applies in other dimensions of life**. Much of our stress and pain comes not from any problem itself, but from our trying to resist the problem and hold on tightly.

● **When we "let go"** — physically, emotionally, inter-personally, spiritually — your increased flexibility often lowers the stress-pain level.

VARIATION

■ This exercise provides a good warm-up to a more complete exploration of relaxation techniques such as *Unwinding (Stress 1, p 73)*.

TRAINER'S NOTES

CONTRIBUTORS

Martha Belknap, MA. Salina Star Route, Gold Hill, Boulder, CO 80302. 303/447-YOGA. Marti is an educational consultant with a specialty in creative relaxation and stress management skills. She has 25 years of teaching experience at all levels. Marti offers relaxation workshops and creativity courses through schools, universities, hospitals and businesses. She is author of **Taming Your Dragons**, *a collection of creative relaxation activities for home and school.*

J J Cochran. Speaker/Trainer, Professional Speakers International, 4022 Pillsbury, Minneapolis, MN 55409. 612/825-8437. J J Cochran, a rare talent, inspires people with concrete, usable ideas. This spirited woman stimulates her audiences' own power so people leave better equipped to face life's challenges. Inspiration, self-esteem and professional power-building are the focus of her 125 annual keynotes/seminars/workshops.

Tim Hatfield, Ph.D. Counselor Education, Winona State University, Winona MN 55987. 507/457-5337. Tim is an educational psychologist whose teaching, workshops and consultation with organizations has focused on stress management and wellness, family and organizational health and lifelong human development issues.

John-Henry Pfifferling, PhD. Director, Center for Professional Well-Being, 5102 Chapel Hill Blvd, Durham NC 27707. 919/489-9167. John-Henry is founder and director of the Center of Professional Well-Being. His PhD in Applied Medical Anthropology and post-doctoral training in Psychiatry and Internal Medicine uniquely qualify him as consultant to professional organizations concerned with preventing impairment. John-Henry specializes in coping skills training for professionals, particularly in medicine.

Sandy Queen. Director, LIFEWORKS, PO Box 2668, Columbia MD 21045. 301/796-5310. Author of **Wellness For Children** *and President of the Organization of Wellness Networks, Sandy maintains a busy practice as an independent health consultant. She is best known in the Washington area for her stress management workshops in business and industry. Sandy was recently appointed to the Maryland State Commission on Physical Fitness.*

Gloria Singer ACSW. Miller Dwan Medical Center, 502 East 2nd St, Duluth MN 55805. 218/720-1305. Gloria's background as a social worker and educator are valuable assets in her position as Employee Assistance Administrator at Miller Dwan Medical Center. In that capacity she has enjoyed designing site-specific programs in stress management and wellness as well as training, counseling and group work with employees and their families.

Mary O'Brien Sippel, RN MS. 1817 Woodland Ave, Duluth MN 55803. 218/723-6130 (work) 218/724-5935 (home). Mary is still one of Whole Person Associates' most enthusiastic faculty. Now a counselor and faculty member at the College of St. Scholastic, Mary continues to inspire others to care for themselves and stay vital. Mary's experience in teaching stress management across the country has enabled her to be her own best caretaker as career woman, wife and mother of two.

Sally Strosahl, MA. Marriage & Family Therapist, 436 Watson, Aurora IL 60505. 312/851-4446. Sally has an MA in clinical psychology; trained at the Wholistic Health Center; researched the relationship between stress and illness. In addition to her private practice in marriage and family therapy, Sally frequently presents workshops in the areas of stress management, burnout, support groups, parenting and combining career and motherhood. She particularly enjoys working with "systems" (family, work groups, agencies, business, churches) to help enhance each member's growth and well-being.

David X Swenson, PhD. Director of Student Development, College of St Scholastica, 1200 Kenwood Ave, Duluth MN 55811. 218/723-6085 (work) 218/724-6903 (home). A licensed consulting psychologist, Dave maintains a private practice in addition to his administrative, educational and therapeutic roles at the college. He provides consultation and training to human services, health and law enforcement agencies.

©1983 Whole Person Press   PO Box 3151 Duluth MN 55812   (218) 728-6807